The End of Epilepsy?

Oxford Medical Histories Series

This series of Oxford Medical Histories is designed to bring to a wide readership of clinical doctors and others from many backgrounds a short but comprehensive text setting out the essentials of differing areas of medicine. Volumes in this series are written by doctors and with doctors, in particular, in mind as the readership.

History describes the knowledge acquired over time by human beings. It is a form of storytelling, of organizing knowledge, of sorting and giving impetus to information. The study of medical history, just like the history of other human endeavours, enables us to analyse our knowledge of the past in order to plan our journey forward and hence try to limit repetition of our mistakes—a sort of planned process of Natural Selection, described as being in the tradition of one of the most famous of medical historians, William Osler. Medical history also encourages and trains us to use an academic approach to our studies which thereby should become more precise, more meaningful, and more productive. Medical history should be enjoyable too, since that is a powerful stimulus to move forward, a fun thing to do both individually and in groups.

The inspiring book that led to this series introduced us to clinical neurology, genetics, and the history of those with muscular dystrophy. Alan and Marcia Emery explored *The History of a Genetic Disease*, now often styled Meryon's disease rather than Duchenne Muscular Dystrophy. The first to describe a disease process is not necessarily the owner of the eponym but the Emerys are helping put that right for their subject, Edward Meryon. The second book in the series, on radiology, took us on a journey round a world of images.

Thus future volumes in this series of Oxford Medical Histories will continue the journey through the history of our bodies, of their relationship to our environment, of the joyful and the sad situations that envelope us from our individual beginnings to our ends. We should travel towards other aspects of our humanity, always leaving us with more questions than answers since each new discovery leads to more questions, exponential sets of issues for us to study, further thoughts and attempts to solve the big questions that surround our existence. Medicine is about people and so is history; the study of the combination of the duo can be very powerful. What do you think?

Christopher Gardner-Thorpe, MD, FRCP, FACP
Series Advisor, Oxford Medical Histories

The End of Epilepsy?
A history of the modern era of epilepsy 1860–2010

Dieter Schmidt
Emeritus Professor of Neurology, Free University Berlin
and Head of Epilepsy Research Group Berlin, Germany

Simon Shorvon
Professor of Neurology, Institute of Neurology, University
College London, and Consultant Neurologist National
Hospital for Neurology and Neurosurgery, London, UK

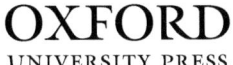

OXFORD
UNIVERSITY PRESS

Great Clarendon Street, Oxford, OX2 6DP,
United Kingdom

Oxford University Press is a department of the University of Oxford.
It furthers the University's objective of excellence in research, scholarship,
and education by publishing worldwide. Oxford is a registered trade mark of
Oxford University Press in the UK and in certain other countries

© Oxford University Press 2016

The moral rights of the authors have been asserted

First Edition published in 2016

Impression: 1

All rights reserved. No part of this publication may be reproduced, stored in
a retrieval system, or transmitted, in any form or by any means, without the
prior permission in writing of Oxford University Press, or as expressly permitted
by law, by licence or under terms agreed with the appropriate reprographics
rights organization. Enquiries concerning reproduction outside the scope of the
above should be sent to the Rights Department, Oxford University Press, at the
address above

You must not circulate this work in any other form
and you must impose this same condition on any acquirer

Published in the United States of America by Oxford University Press
198 Madison Avenue, New York, NY 10016, United States of America

British Library Cataloguing in Publication Data
Data available

Library of Congress Control Number: 2016943985

ISBN 978-0-19-872590-9

Printed and bound by
CPI Group (UK) Ltd, Croydon, CR0 4YY

Oxford University Press makes no representation, express or implied, that the
drug dosages in this book are correct. Readers must therefore always check
the product information and clinical procedures with the most up-to-date
published product information and data sheets provided by the manufacturers
and the most recent codes of conduct and safety regulations. The authors and
the publishers do not accept responsibility or legal liability for any errors in the
text or for the misuse or misapplication of material in this work. Except where
otherwise stated, drug dosages and recommendations are for the non-pregnant
adult who is not breast-feeding

Links to third party websites are provided by Oxford in good faith and
for information only. Oxford disclaims any responsibility for the materials
contained in any third party website referenced in this work.

Foreword

> If there's any illness for which people offer many remedies, you may be sure that particular illness is incurable, I think.
>
> Anton Checkov, *The Cherry Orchard*, 1904, tr. Julius West, 1916. In: *Plays by Anton Checkov*, 2nd series. New York: Scribner's, 1917

Worldwide, roughly 1% of all people suffer from epilepsy. It is a common disease of the brain, and although repeating epileptic seizures are its clinical hallmark, the condition amounts to more than just having seizures. Physical and psychological co-morbidities, personality disturbances, issues of self-esteem and confidence, neurological deficits, intellectual impairment, and other non-neurological conditions keep company with seizures in some patients, and when seizures cannot be controlled, there is also a small risk of premature death. Furthermore, epilepsy is not just a medical phenomenon, but a social construct, with cultural, political, and financial consequences. People with epilepsy are exposed to stigma and burdened with disadvantages which can be more far reaching than the epileptic seizures themselves. There are indeed many remedies, but as Chekhov rightly surmised, no cure.

Nevertheless, progress has been made in recent times through clinical and scientific research. On all fronts, epilepsy has been intensively studied, and in the last 50 years for instance, around 200 000 articles are listed in the scientific literature with epilepsy or epileptic seizures as a main theme. Epilepsy is also much discussed in general media and makes its presence felt in many areas of human activity. Much has been achieved and impressive scientific advances have been made. However, one might think that as a result of this activity we would now have an understanding of the fundamentals of condition, for instance about how and why the epilepsies develop, or would have discovered better methods of preventing the condition or evolved greatly improved approaches to its treatment. Yet, in reality, despite best efforts, over 100 years of epilepsy research has achieved somewhat less than might have been expected, and less than is often proclaimed. Epilepsy, which in 1860 was in the forefront of neurological research and theory, has been overtaken by progress in other neurological conditions and it has been overshadowed.

Indeed, despite the billions of dollars spent on epilepsy medical care and research, it could be argued that the most impressive improvements are not medical or scientific, but rather are found in the better societal attitudes towards people with epilepsy, the reduction of stigma, and their better social integration.

Epilepsy, like the Roman god Janus,[1] presents a dark side for many patients. Current drugs aim to suppress seizures and are palliative at best, but seem to do nothing to alter the progression of the disease, and the same applies to therapeutic devices. Furthermore, even the best therapies do not control seizures in 20% of cases, and the antiepileptic drugs come with side effects in many people. Although several initially promising agents were developed with the aim of preventing the disease in those at risk, successive experimental trials have failed. The basic mechanisms of epilepsy and its treatment remain only very incompletely explained, despite intensive modern molecular and physiological research, and research strategies for the discovery of antiseizure drugs that did not work 50 years ago are still being pursued up to this day. Industry (and not so much academia or institutions of government) has identified a dizzying variety of new treatments for seizures, but these are effective in only selected cases. Surgery of the brain can control seizures when drugs have failed, but itself is destructive and risky and is sometimes futile, leaving the victim damaged. Advanced treatments are not available in many parts of the world. The enormous achievements of neuroimaging and other investigatory modalities have, with a few laudable exceptions, not resulted in substantially novel therapy or more effective surgical treatment of focal epilepsies. Political, financial, and societal influences impact on patients' lives, mostly negatively.

Why is this book written? It may be easiest to point out right at the start what this book is not about. Don't expect another medical tome on epilepsy for those who want to know the medical practicalities of managing epilepsy in the clinic or a lay guide to, or description of, the condition. Nor is this a complete historical survey of modern epilepsy, which would not be possible in a book of this size. Do not expect either, a scientific review. This is not the purpose of our narrative, and for this reason, nor do we provide extensive reference to the literature. Whilst we trust that the book is sufficiently scholarly, that the facts asserted are accurate, it remains at its heart an expression of our personal perspectives. We are interested in exploring the anatomy of success and failure in epilepsy research and in epilepsy care. With this in mind, the book takes the form of what are essentially a series of reflections, focusing as much on what has not been achieved as what has, and has been written with two main objectives:

1. To provide a *biography of modern epilepsy* in the form of a brief and selective narrative of some of the important developments in epilepsy research, with its many ups and downs, over the period since 1860 (especially in

Chapters 1-5). We have focused on the medical not the societal aspects, though have tried to incorporate some impressions also of the latter. We chose 1860 as our starting point as this can be considered to be the dawn of the 'modern era' of epilepsy; a period which began with John Hughlings Jackson's definition of epilepsy, the discovery of bromide therapy, the birth of neurosurgery, and the rise of modern science.

The history of epilepsy up until this period is well covered in Owsei Temkin's outstanding and scholarly book *The Falling Sickness* (2), published first in 1945 and then in a revised edition in 1971. The last section of Temkin's book is subtitled 'The age of Hughlings Jackson' and the last chapter in this section is entitled 'The end of falling sickness?'. Temkin hoped, with the advance of science and of culture, that epilepsy might cease to be 'a paradigm of the suffering of both body and soul in disease'. He was referring as much to the cultural as to the medical impact of epilepsy, and the great value of his approach was his vision of epilepsy as a fundamentally social as well as medical phenomenon. Obviously, and with a heavy dose of hindsight, we know now that the concept of the end of epilepsy, which seemed possible for him to contemplate, has proved too optimistic. Epilepsy has sadly not become extinct and suffering of body and soul remain. We chose our book title from Temkin's last chapter, and have attempted to expand on some of the themes he proposed. Temkin considered that an ideal history was one: 'which finds a synthesis of the somatic and psychological, the individual and social factors; … and is more than a record of its coming and going, of its clinical manifestations, of the impressions it made upon man; … [and is] a blend of its natural history … and its human history'. He considered that it was not possible at the time of writing to extend his history beyond the age of Jackson.

A further 50 years have passed, and still much is in flux, and as Temkin was, so are we also too close to modern events to provide a definitive perspective of contemporary science. Nevertheless, it is clear that there are overarching themes which underlie the modern history of epilepsy, and we emphasise these to give meaning to the narrative and prevent the book simply being a list of events and dates. These themes include: that science proceeds erratically, that all is not progress, and there have been many medical 'culs-de-sac'; the concepts of disease and its treatment are not objective, and there is a major societal impact on all aspects of medicine; medical advances are not necessarily hypothesis based, but are driven also by personality, societal influence, and technological advances; chance place a part, and wrong hypotheses are proposed—yet the drug works; the agenda of scientific research is complex and the aim is not simply the advance of knowledge; the patient is in the middle of a chaotic whirlpool of competing interests.

Our biography of epilepsy is therefore, inevitably in this short book, selective, and the reader is referred to other histories of epilepsy and its treatment in the twentieth century for more detail, although none have the breadth or reach of Temkin.[2]

2. Our second objective is to provide a *critical look* at where we are today, and how we got here. We have decided to take a deliberately sceptical, and occasionally heretical, perspective and direct our focus particularly onto the negative aspects of this history and our current position (especially in Chapters 6-8). Carl Sagan wrote that sceptical scrutiny is the means by which deep thoughts can be winnowed from deep nonsense. He was writing about science and religion, and saw the link between the objective and the subjective. In epilepsy, there have been deep thoughts and great improvements, but there has also been deep nonsense. We have therefore included deliberately, the dark side of the story of modern epilepsy, which is less often presented and do not apologise for this. We see it as important to articulate these less satisfactory aspects of the history as an antidote to the anodyne and uncritical reporting that is commonplace in our world. All is not perfect, and progress in science is not, as is commonly portrayed, an inexorable and incremental journey to the stars. If you think about it, it is quite surprising that we have not been able to remove epilepsy from the long list of serious and intractable brain disorders, given the billions of dollars and the best medical efforts to develop more effective epilepsy drugs and to improve the outcome of epilepsy surgery. Social and political influences have clouded progress, and science has meandered up many blind alleys, wasting time and opportunity. Financial considerations have weighed heavily on our story, with industry as much as science calling the tune. We have tried to make an effort to separate the wheat from the chaff in the development of better epilepsy care. Events and concepts of historic consequence are discussed and we have left out minor discoveries of little longer-term significance.

Another warning. In this work, we express our personal opinions which may be sometimes at variance with mainstream thought. We emphasise that we certainly to do not want to offend any in the epilepsy field by taking different positions, and apologise in advance if we do so, but we honestly believe that by being forthright in our opinions we may encourage fresh thinking and new debate, and that this approach can be only good for epilepsy. We do not blandly evade controversial topics in our book and fully respect if people disagree or do not like our approach. We believe deeply in the value of intellectual argument and debate.

The book has taken a largely medical perspective, and we have emphasised particularly therapy, as treatment and cure are the ultimate purposes of medicine.

Chapter 1 considers the question of what epilepsy really is and Chapter 2 its societal meaning and consequences for, as both chapters try to make clear, despite our medical perspective, epilepsy is certainly not 'just a medical disease'. The point is also made that the societal impact of epilepsy (*being epileptic*) is for many patients more onerous than the medical consequences of epilepsy (*having epilepsy*). Chapters 3–5 outline events in the evolution of the drug and surgical treatment of epilepsy, in the form of a narrative history emphasising the erratic nature of progress and both the importance of science and particularly of luck in the process of drug discovery. We have stressed the influence of fashion and societal attitudes on science and medicine, and the role of industry and its flip-side regulation. We are throughout interested to capture creative moments in epilepsy care and examine how exactly important progress in the treatment of epilepsy developed and how it was derailed despite the best intentions of very bright people. Chapters 6 and 7 discuss the 'dark side' of epilepsy, directing attention on to the deficiencies of our assessment of drug treatment, low-quality care, and various failed medical theories of epilepsy. We outline the achievements and lost opportunities of the formal structures and bureaucracies of epilepsy, and how their rigidity is the enemy of progress. Our purpose is to point to the fragilities and fashion inherent in our systems, and to guard against the too easy complacency. Chapter 8 muses on the future and the ways in which the *End of Epilepsy* might in fact be realised.

Our spotlight on the dark side results in less attention on the many aspects of progress made in the field in our period than may be considered justified. We realise that this is the case, but the celebration of myriad successes is not the primary point of the book. This biography doesn't romanticise the bright side of epilepsy, for instance the fact that epilepsy is for many patients a passing disease that can be well dealt with. We generally have looked into the shadows, and cannot ignore what is for many, the dread of having a serious and life-threatening condition imposing suffering and distress. We have to acknowledge that, although the end of epilepsy is in reach of some, there is, at present, no prescribed scientific path to the end of epilepsy for others. Regardless of the severity of epilepsy, patients, with the support of their physicians and modern medicine, must create their own solutions to the multiple issues they face.

Notes

1. Interestingly, Owsei Temkin was himself interested in the analogy of Janus and wrote a collection of essays entitled *The Double Face of Janus and Other Essays in the History of Medicine* (1).
2. Examples of modern histories of epilepsy, which form source material for this book, include Friedlander (3), Lennox and Lennox (4), Shorvon et al. (5), and Shorvon (6). Although our book title is based on Temkin, we notice too that Lennox and Lennox

(4) finished their two-volume work with 'May what is written help to succor those in need and aid the efforts of those who will open the way to the common end, the End of Epilepsy'.

References

1. **Temkin O.** *The Double Face of Janus and Other Essays in the History of Medicine.* Baltimore, MD: Johns Hopkins Press; 2006.
2. **Temkin O.** *The Falling Sickness: A History of Epilepsy from the Greeks to the Beginnings of Modern Neurology.* Baltimore, MD: Johns Hopkins University Press; 1945.
3. **Friedlander WJ.** *History of Modern Epilepsy: The Beginning, 1865–1914.* Westport, CT: Greenwood Press; 2001.
4. **Lennox WG, Lennox M.** *Epilepsy and Related Disorders.* Boston, MA: Little Brown; 1960.
5. **Shorvon SD, Weiss G, Avanzini G, et al.** *International League Against Epilepsy 1909-2009: a centenary history.* Oxford: Wiley-Blackwell; 2009.
6. **Shorvon SD, Weiss G, Wolf P, Andermann F** (eds). To celebrate the centenary of Epilepsia and the ILAE: aspects of the history of epilepsy 1909–2009. *Epilepsia* 2009; 50(Suppl 3):1–151.
7. **Shorvon SD.** Historical introduction. In: The drug treatment of epilepsy from 1857–2015. In: Shorvon S, Perucca E, Engel J (eds). *The Treatment of Epilepsy*, 4th ed. Oxford: Wiley Blackwell; 2015:i–xxiii.
8. **Shorvon SD.** Historical introduction: the causes of epilepsy in the pre-molecular era (1860–1960). In: Shorvon SD, Andermann F, Guerrini R (eds) *The Causes of Epilepsy: Common and Uncommon Causes in Adults and Children.* Cambridge: Cambridge University Press; 2011:1–20.

Contents

Abbreviations *xiii*

1 What is Epilepsy? *1*

2 Attitudes *21*

3 The Pharmaceutical Phoenix Rises *39*

4 Modern Blockbusters *61*

5 Resecting Epilepsy *81*

6 The Dark Side of Epilepsy *107*

7 Culs-de-Sac and Bureaucracies *127*

8 Is the End of Epilepsy in Sight? *155*

Appendix: Dating Epilepsy *173*

Index *179*

Abbreviations

3D	three-dimensional		MES	maximal electric shock
CNS	central nervous system		NINDS	National Institute of Neurological Disorders and Stroke
CT	computed tomography			
EMA	European Medicines Agency		PDS	paroxysmal depolarisation shift
FDA	Food and Drug Administration		PTZ	pentylenetetrazole
GABA	gamma-aminobutyric acid		STM	science, technology, and medicine
IBE	International Bureau for Epilepsy			
ILAE	International League Against Epilepsy		SPECT	single-positron emission computed tomography
			SUDEP	sudden unexplained death in epilepsy
LBS	levetiracetam binding site			
MRI	magnetic resonance imaging		WHO	World Health Organization

Chapter 1

What is Epilepsy?

What is epilepsy? This is not an easy question largely because it is a phenomenon that does not exist in a vacuum, it affects people who have historical and geographical location, and is more than just a physical condition, the fact of simply having epileptic seizures, and is more than a simple medical entity. It is, as Temkin (Figure 1.1) put it, a tangle of 'human history and natural history' (1). It has cultural, geographic, and historical meanings and significances well beyond the walls of the neurological citadel, and these defy a single perspective. Oliver Wendell Homes, cited by Temkin, wrote: 'If I wished to show a student the difficulties of getting at truth from medical experience, I would give him the history of epilepsy to read' (2). We concur with this sentiment and the complexities of the condition are one theme which runs through this short book (Figure 1.2).

But, let us start at the beginning. The first manuscript on epilepsy was entitled 'On the Sacred Disease' and this was a collection of Hippocratic writings from around the year 400 BC.[1] This text attacks the conjecture, then widely held by the credulous populace, that epilepsy was a divine or magical disease, and a fit was the result of bodily possession by demons, evil or divine spirits. The Hippocratic manuscript stated that epilepsy was a disease of the brain and, like other physical diseases, could be treated by diet and drugs. It firmly located epilepsy in the brain, for the first time in recorded history, and staked a claim for it being a physical 'disease' explicable in terms of natural science. This ran counter to the contemporary medical folklore, but this idea was lost in the medieval period, and disputes about the nature, location, and significance of epilepsy have continued ever since.

What is an Epileptic Seizure?

The focus of our book is the modern era, starting with the work of John Hughlings Jackson in London in the 1860s–1890s, and it is with Jackson that the first modern understanding of seizures begins (Figure 1.3). It was with quite astonishing prescience that Jackson wrote in 1870 (3): 'a convulsion is but a symptom, and implies only that there is an occasional, an excessive, and a disorderly discharge of nerve tissue on muscles'. And in 1873 (4), he also added

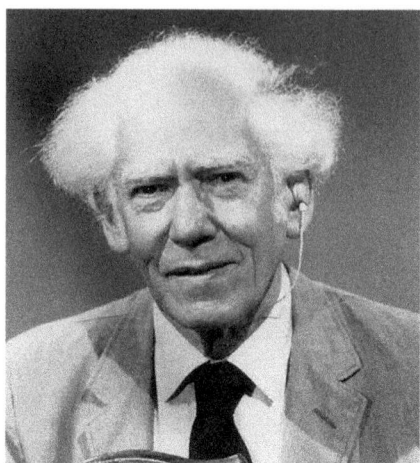

Figure 1.1 Owsei Temkin (1902–2002), born in Russia, was Professor of the History of Medicine at Johns Hopkins University. His book, *The Falling Sickness*, is the definitive scholarly work on the history of epilepsy.
Reproduced with permission from The Johns Hopkins Medical Institutions. Copyright © 2016 The Johns Hopkins Medical Institutions, The Johns Hopkins University. All rights reserved.

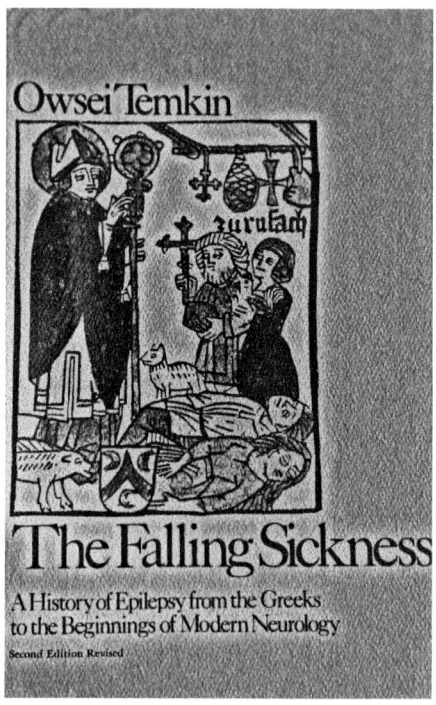

Figure 1.2 Front cover of *The Falling Sickness* by Owsei Temkin.
Reproduced with permission from The Johns Hopkins Medical Institutions. Copyright © 2016 The Johns Hopkins Medical Institutions, The Johns Hopkins University. All rights reserved.

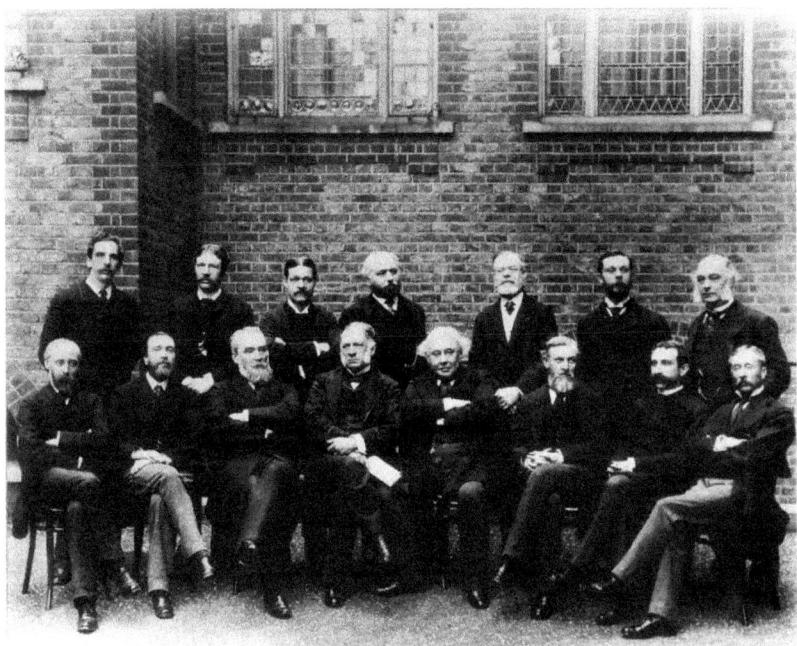

Figure 1.3 A staff portrait at the National Hospital for the Relief and Cure of the Paralysed and the Epileptic in 1886. In the front row, John Hughlings Jackson is third from the left, William Gowers is sixth from the left, and David Ferrier is at the right-hand end. Victor Horsley is standing at the end of the back row on the right. Reproduced by kind permission of the Queen Square Library, Archive, and Museum, London.

cerebral localisation to his definition: 'Epilepsy is the name for occasional, sudden, excessive, rapid and local discharges of grey matter' (Figure 1.4). Jackson's postulation that a seizure was a cortical 'discharge' was an extraordinary insight based as it was entirely on his observations of the clinical features of seizures. His theory that the physiological disturbance of epilepsy was located in the grey matter of the brain was also revolutionary at a time when most contemporaries (and indeed Jackson himself at the beginning of his career) placed the seat of some epilepsies as some sort of reflex in the deeper parts of the brain, the medulla, or the spinal cord. He considered the 'excessive discharge' to be chemical in nature. To Jackson, a convulsion was a 'physiological fulminate, like the gunpowder in a cannon' and just as gunpowder can store energy that is liberated when firing the gun, so the energy stored in nerve cells could be explosively liberated in an epileptic discharge. He held that the abnormal levels of stored energy were due to deranged 'nutrition', and that this in turn was due usually to congestion of small blood vessels.[2] Switch the

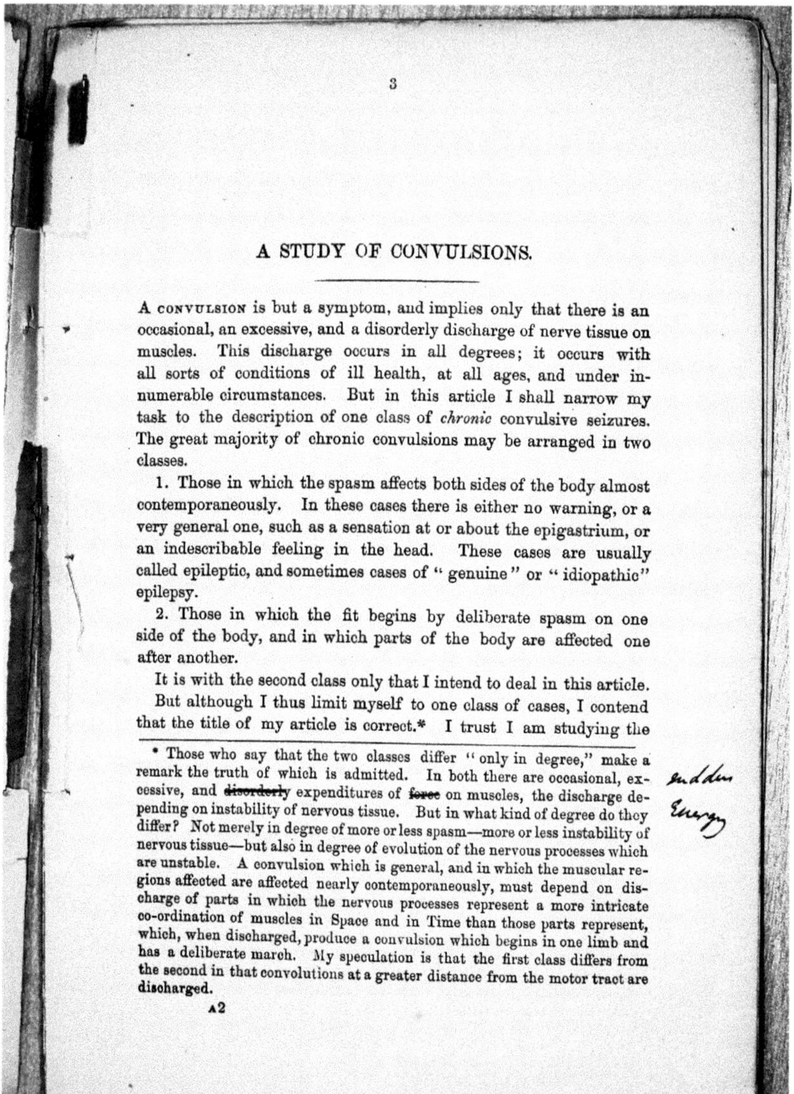

A STUDY OF CONVULSIONS.

A CONVULSION is but a symptom, and implies only that there is an occasional, an excessive, and a disorderly discharge of nerve tissue on muscles. This discharge occurs in all degrees; it occurs with all sorts of conditions of ill health, at all ages, and under innumerable circumstances. But in this article I shall narrow my task to the description of one class of *chronic* convulsive seizures. The great majority of chronic convulsions may be arranged in two classes.

1. Those in which the spasm affects both sides of the body almost contemporaneously. In these cases there is either no warning, or a very general one, such as a sensation at or about the epigastrium, or an indescribable feeling in the head. These cases are usually called epileptic, and sometimes cases of " genuine " or " idiopathic " epilepsy.

2. Those in which the fit begins by deliberate spasm on one side of the body, and in which parts of the body are affected one after another.

It is with the second class only that I intend to deal in this article.

But although I thus limit myself to one class of cases, I contend that the title of my article is correct.* I trust I am studying the

---

* Those who say that the two classes differ " only in degree," make a remark the truth of which is admitted. In both there are occasional, excessive, and ~~disorderly~~ expenditures of ~~force~~ on muscles, the discharge depending on instability of nervous tissue. But in what kind of degree do they differ? Not merely in degree of more or less spasm—more or less instability of nervous tissue—but also in degree of evolution of the nervous processes which are unstable. A convulsion which is general, and in which the muscular regions affected are nearly contemporaneously, must depend on discharge of parts in which the nervous processes represent a more intricate co-ordination of muscles in Space and in Time than those parts represent, which, when discharged, produce a convulsion which begins in one limb and has a deliberate march. My speculation is that the first class differs from the second in that convulsions at a greater distance from the motor tract are discharged.

[margin note: *sudden Energy*]

Figure 1.4 John Hughlings Jackson's own copy of 'A study of convulsions' published in the *Transactions of the St Andrews Medical Graduates Association*, 1869, 1870, 3:162–204. This shows the first version of Jackson's definition of a convulsion and his own handwritten revisions
Reproduced by kind permission of the Queen Square Library, Archive, and Museum, London.

word 'nutrition' to 'neurotransmission' and Jackson's framework is the same as our own. Jackson also recognised that there were different types of seizures and that the clinical form of the seizure depended on the exact localisation of the excessive discharge. The paradigmatic type was what is now called the 'Jacksonian seizure' (a term coined by Charcot[3]) which arises in the central cortex, and this fitted in to his view of the somatotropic representation of the body in the nervous system. He recognised that the onset of the fit (i.e. of the sudden excessive discharge) would give away its location, and as he wrote in 1868, 'One of the most important questions we can ask an epileptic patient is "How does the fit begin?"', and in 1873, 'There is nothing more important than to note where a convulsion begins, for the inference is that the first motor symptom is the sign of the beginning of the central discharge', and 'The mode of onset is the most important matter in the anatomical investigation of any case of epilepsy'. This was all magnificent and singular theory, which placed Jackson at the head of nineteenth-century neuroscience, and through these ideas, he had moved epilepsy into the scientific age, and changed entirely the conceptual framework of the disease. His theories have stood the test of time, and remain at the core of the mechanistic ideas of epilepsy and medical definitions of an epileptic seizure which we still hold today more than 150 years later.

The most important next historical step in our thinking about a 'seizure' was the introduction of the electroencephalogram (EEG) into clinical practice in the 1940s. The EEG is a test of 'function', not structure, and offers the promise of being able to identify, visualise, and measure the 'abnormal discharge'. With the advent of the EEG came the recognition that some seizures were indeed localised as Jackson had shown, but that others seemed to affect simultaneously wide areas of cortex in both cerebral hemispheres. This became a fundamental dichotomy and led to a classification of epileptic seizures into focal (partial) and generalised types. The distinction between partial and generalised seizures has become controversial in recent years, as it is increasingly recognised that a neural network underpins many apparently focal seizures, and conversely that many generalised seizures have in fact 'focal' elements. The concept of a 'focus' is now thought simplistic, and the emphasis has shifted to a more sophisticated 'systems' view of the nature of a seizure.

It might also be thought that the EEG, by allowing the visualisation of the 'excessive discharge', would clarify what is a seizure and what is not. However, as is almost always the case when a new technology is applied to medicine, the situation is more complex than originally conceived. The EEG in fact has complicated the issue of definition, and by providing a 'window' on the electrical activity of the brain has demonstrated a grey area between a seizure and non-seizure state. For a start, there are abnormalities on the EEG which occur in the absence of a seizure, the so-called interictal abnormalities, but these have shown sometimes to be associated with very brief and very subtle impairments of function and so in some senses these themselves might be classified as seizures. Conversely, limbic EEG studies have demonstrated 'epileptiform' discharges at times when an individual is experiencing emotional or psychotic symptoms, even in people without a history of epilepsy, and with a normal scalp EEG—should these be considered seizures? (5). Sometimes, EEG activity, indistinguishable from seizure activity, also occurs in the absence of any symptoms, and sometimes seizures occur without any obvious alteration in the EEG from the interictal state, for instance, in some cases of West syndrome or in neonatal seizures. Finally, it should not be forgotten that the EEG is the result of summation of the potentials of a large number of neurons close to the recording electrode, and is therefore inherently a relatively blunt instrument, and that what is going on in any individual cell is beyond its capacity of resolution.

The cellular mechanisms of the 'excessive discharge' (the epileptic seizures) have been the subject of intense scientific study, several Nobel Prizes have been awarded for work in related areas, and today a working knowledge of the details of the physiology and chemistry of the seizure discharge has been gained.[4] A seizure is recognised to be the manifestation of synchronised excessive discharges from groups of neurons, caused by changes in electrical thresholds, neurotransmitters, and chemical fluxes through ion channels and other chemical pathways. Physiologically, the hallmark of epilepsy is the so-called paroxysmal depolarisation shift (PDS) which is a cellular phenomenon rendering individual cells hyperexcitable. The normal electrical activity of a cell is superseded by fast, repetitive, and disproportionately large electrical movements which result in violent contractions of muscles and disturbances of sensations, consciousness, and mentation ('excessive and disorderly discharges of nerve tissue on muscles' much as Jackson predicted). This activity overwhelms the natural inhibitory processes of the brain and has a tendency to activate simultaneously neuronal networks in the brain or to spread like a wave through neighbouring or connected brain areas. The detailed chemistry and physiology of a seizure discharge have been well studied in slices of brain observed under the microscope, and in animal models *in vivo* and *in vitro*, and the conditions which initiate and terminate a seizure are to some extent now known.

The unravelling of the chemical and physical nature of the epileptic seizure is one of the triumphs of the modern era in epilepsy. The scientific explanation of an epileptic seizure has led to targeted approaches to treatment and has laid to rest the idea that a seizure is a manifestation of possession or some other supernatural phenomenon. Seizures have to a large extent been 'demystified' and although much still remains to be discovered, particularly in terms of the nature of the neural networks and systems, we are over the hump when it comes to understanding seizures. However, the same is not true of 'epilepsy'.

What is Epilepsy?

Jackson wrote that the convulsion was 'but a symptom' and recognised that the definition of epilepsy was more difficult. Lennox,[5] who represented the advanced medical viewpoint in 1960, reiterated what Jackson wrote and stated that 'the fits are the symptoms, and the epilepsies are the diseases' and that what makes epilepsy a 'disease' is the fact that it has a 'cause'. This is the strictly medical model of disease, and the emphasis on cause avoids any circular arguments about definition which in fact have plagued later classifications. Lennox, and Jackson, and indeed all other writers on this topic, noted that there are myriad causes which can be structural or biochemical, or genetic or developmental, and may or may not be demonstrable. The cases where no cause can be identified are labelled as 'idiopathic' or 'cryptogenic'; these terms imply not that there is no cause, just that the cause has eluded detection. Absence of evidence is not evidence of absence.

In this medical model of disease, therefore, the emphasis on cause is fundamental, but in the case of epilepsy, establishing a cause is not necessarily an easy matter.[6] Again, there are complexities and a number of hurdles that prevent easy definition of cause. One is the indubitable fact that the production of seizures is usually a multifactorial process, dependent on the interplay of constitutional and acquired factors. The constitutional influence is itself the result both of an individual's genetics and also of the processes of brain development, and the acquired factors include the presence of brain lesions and also 'triggering' factors from the environment (alcohol, lack of sleep, stress, etc.). This is a complex brew, and choosing one element as 'the cause' of an epilepsy can never be wholly precise (the same applies to many human characteristics—height and weight, for instance). Obviously in some cases, there is a strongly predominant cause, the presence of a brain tumour for instance, which may dwarf the others in importance, but in many cases, the extent to which any individual factor predominates is not necessarily very obvious. A good example is the individual with idiopathic generalised epilepsy who only has seizures when sleep deprived. Is the major 'cause' genetic (but no gene has been identified), developmental (but no developmental anomaly is identified), or environmental (i.e. sleep deprivation)? We do not think it is possible logically to say.

Another important issue, raised first by Jackson, is the level at which 'cause' is decided. We commonly consider 'downstream' pathologies to be the 'cause' (Jackson called these the 'remote' causes), such as the brain tumour, the sleep deprivation, or the genetic make-up. However, one could equally consider the cause to be the final molecular mechanism of the seizure itself (Jackson called this the primary, or physiological, cause). Think of the analogy of a flood—is it due to the rainstorms in the hills or the inadequate height of the river embankment walls? In other words, where in the chain of causation, can the blame for the seizure be pinned? Again, we do not think there is a single answer to this quandary. Furthermore, Jackson also suggested that different remote causes might result in the same physiological change, which is the 'fundamental' cause. This view of 'cause' as being 'causal mechanism' seems to us to be of great importance and often not given due appreciation. To what extent different pathologies produce the same causal mechanisms is something upon which future research should focus.

Another complication in the assignment of cause in any individual's epilepsy is the fact that the epilepsy evolves over time and what precipitates a seizure at the onset of the condition is not necessarily the same as in chronic epilepsy. Epilepsy, in other words, is itself a dynamic process. All these points were recognised by the leading neurologists in the nineteenth century but have tended to be ignored in more recent times. One approach is to try to express causal factors in terms of their statistical weight (for instance, by calculating 'odds ratios' or 'susceptibilities'), and this makes sense although often available data are insufficient to achieve this.

The medical model of disease though is just one side of the coin. The idea of 'disease' has much more extensive connotations, and this particularly applies to epilepsy; a point emphasised by Temkin who considered epilepsy to be 'a paradigm of the suffering of both body and soul in disease'. The social and cultural connotations of epilepsy can often be far more important than the occurrence of seizures. In other words, having epilepsy is far more than just *having seizures*. There are impacts on social interactions, social relationships, marriage, domestic life, education, and employment. There are issues of dependency and identity, self-esteem, and self-confidence. These dominate the lives of many patients. Although based on the occurrence of seizures, these aspects transcend the seizures. Seizures may occur typically once every few months and last a few minutes, but what has been described as 'being epileptic' is a permanent internal (existential) state of being, a psychic position, which persists sometimes years after the end of the seizures. There are few conditions in which the disconnect between the symptoms and the disease state is so massive.

There is also a societal perspective on the condition, which has great implications for the sufferer. The manifestations of the disease are at one level just the seizures, but societal reactions to, and interactions with, the person with epilepsy often transcend a narrow concern with seizures, and involve legislative and attitudinal elements which are all-persuasive. The position of a person with epilepsy is hugely influenced by the cultural norms of the time and by geographical location; and it is for this reason that any satisfactory definition of epilepsy must be a blend of its natural and human histories. As we show in Chapter 2, the societal attitude to epilepsy is very much part of its dark side and yet is also perhaps the aspect which has improved most in the modern era.

Definition in mental disease (and in this sense, this includes epilepsy, as it is a manifestation of brain activity) is a particular issue.[7] Indeed, one strand of socio-political thought raises doubts about the very existence of 'disease' in this sphere, considering the diseases to be mainly, or at least to an extent, social constructs; and they have a point. For instance, much has been recently written about the crude commercialism of symptoms, and the attempts of the pharmaceutical industry to label types of human behaviour as diseases so that they can sell their products as treatment and there can be no doubt that economic and commercial considerations weigh in heavily on disease definitions. Actually, this is not new, and there is a long history of quacks from the medieval period onwards doing exactly the same thing. Others consider the medicalisation of psychological conditions as a technique of imposing social control. As Ivan Illich, a most trenchant critic of the medical model, wrote: 'each civilisation defines its own diseases. What is sickness in one might be chromosomal abnormality, crime, holiness or sin in another' (10). He recognised that being labelled ill is better than being considered a criminal or political deviant, and that the illness role implies that the sufferer is 'an innocent victim of biological mechanisms' rather than being simply lazy, greedy, or a deserter of a social struggle over the 'tools of production'. To Illich, therefore, illness is a social transaction. He has a point, and views on epilepsy historically have exhibited all of these features. Much as the Hippocratic physicians also realised, social attitudes, cultural beliefs, and economic and political realities are as important an influence of what is accepted as illness or disease by society as any physiological attribute.

Of course, it is easier to take a narrower medical view and fall back on definitions which rely on the physiological signature of the epileptic seizures. Even from this perspective, however, the 'idiopathic' diseases in the arena of neurological and psychiatric diseases, including idiopathic epilepsy, are where distinctions between health and disease are most blurred. The rise of the science of genetics creates further difficulties, now in the age of molecular genetics, than it did in the past. It has been long known that genetic variation can confer 'susceptibility' to disease in some people (actually, this is an obvious truism for all our characteristics are to an extent the product of our genes), but modern genetics now provides the tools to be able to begin to identify the molecular nature of polymorphisms associated with susceptibility. However, the susceptibility conferred by genetic variations is often small, and much influenced by epigenetic and epistatic factors.[8] Furthermore, many unaffected people exist who carry these genetic variants, and even if genetic 'defects' do exist in a genome, this does not automatically require categorisation of disease or result in the need for 'treatment'. There are fundamental issues which skate on the thin ice surrounding human rights and human identity, about how society should be tolerant of differences (as Bateson[9] put it, society should treasure its exceptions), how personal identity is formed, and about how to balance an individual's rights against extra cost to society. Epilepsy is now, and has been in the past, strongly bound up in all these considerations. As we explore in Chapter 2, the social impact of epilepsy is in many ways much greater than the simple occurrence of seizures.

Another issue concerns the concept of disability, and its distinction from disease. Jackie Scully (14)[10] has raised various issues which are relevant to epilepsy. She points out that until recently, disability was seen as a medical concept, a 'nominative pathology: a disease, degeneration, defect or deficit located in an individual, and defined by a deviation from a biomedical norm'. She points out though, that there is a distinction to be made between the impairment (say, having fits) and the social, economic, and political reaction (say, banning marriage or driving). The impairment may form an important element in a person's identity and if the disabling elements are taken away, the person is no longer the person he/she was. Scully considers that treating disability can be seen sometimes as violence inflicted on the person, and there are and have been through its recent history many examples of this in epilepsy; this is part of the dark side we will discuss later in this book. Assuming that all idiopathic disease is genetic is another way that harm can be caused, because the phenotype bears a complex relationship to genotype, and to ignore the non-genetic factors influencing this relationship (environmental, developmental, epigenetic, and epistatic) is to grossly oversimplify. As Scully (13, p.653) puts it:

> What ought to concern us about disease and disability is the disadvantage, pain or suffering involved, and in a sense the impairment is always a kind of surrogate marker for this experience. By defining disease or disability in terms of genetic loci, the relationship to experience is made a step more distant: removed not just from the lived experience of the phenotype, but from the development of the phenotype itself. Of course the size of this separation depends on the condition, and in many cases makes no real difference: it would be both stupid and offensive to suggest the need to examine lived experience before deciding that having familial colon cancer entails suffering. Nevertheless, for a lot of conditions (and epilepsy is a paradigmatic example) that at the moment are called disabilities, and bundled together with more easily definable diseases, the situation is not so simple. One take-home message here is that, although disease and disability are regularly lumped together, conflating them is often misleading. Another is that science never simply reflects cultural understandings; it

simultaneously helps craft the definitions as well. Choices of such mundane things as disease models and diagnostic criteria, then, are not just about research agendas or commercial influences. At their heart they embody profound ethical debates about identity, human rights, and the tolerance of difference.

This, we feel, is very well said.

It could be argued that none of this is a concern of science, which is value free and aims only to answer precisely defined questions by scientific experimentation. For those taking this position, science seeks to uncover the true disease mechanisms (including genetic mechanisms), and should not meander into the broader fields of ethics and particularly sociology; it is for others to incorporate these into social or health service structures. In our opinion, this is an arrogant view, with potentially profoundly negative consequences, for scientists, like all others, have a responsibility and duty to society, and no science should ignore its cultural framework. The extreme example of the difficulties such complacency confers, was the pathological work done by Hallervorden and others on the brains of children killed by the Nazis,[11] and even now it is not clear what the ethical position is of accepting or building on the scientific findings in this work. Furthermore, scientific theory or findings are often false or inaccurate (and occasionally deliberate fraud) and the story of epilepsy not free of such mistakes (see Chapter 6). The public and society are at risk of being effectively duped by overhype, faulty conclusions, and vacuous speculation; this happens today in much of genetic and pharmaceutical medicine in the field of epilepsy.

The International League Against Epilepsy Definitions

Over the years, many have proposed definitions and classifications of epilepsy and epileptic seizures. In fact, as these are essentially matters of individual opinion, usually without supporting data, it is always open season in this particular hunt. It is difficult to find an area where so many opinions and such few data exist.

The International League Against Epilepsy (ILAE) is the leading professional association of doctors in the field of epilepsy. It has been in existence since 1909 (with interruptions) and perhaps its most important achievement was its work in the field of classification (work which today is in danger of unravelling) with schemata which are firmly based within the medical model of disease.[12] All definitions have had at their minimum the occurrence of an epileptic seizure, the primary symptom of epilepsy, but there have been interesting variations on the theme and changes of emphasis. The ILAE's first foray into this area was in the publication of the 1973 World Health Organization's (WHO's) 'Glossary of Terms'. In this, epilepsy was defined as a 'chronic brain disorder of various aetiologies characterised by recurrent seizures due to excessive discharges of cerebral neurons, associated with a variety of clinical and laboratory manifestations', and in 2001, the revised glossary defined epilepsy as 'A chronic neurologic condition characterised by recurrent epileptic seizures' and a seizure as 'A manifestation of epileptic (excessive and/or hypersynchronous), usually self-limited activity of neurons in the brain'. These definitions are Jacksonian in origin and became widely accepted, albeit within the narrow confines of the medical model. However, the temptation to change definitions has proved irresistible. In 2006, another ILAE definition of epilepsy was proposed, as 'a disorder of the brain characterised by an enduring predisposition to generate epileptic seizures and by the neurobiological, cognitive, psychological and social consequences of this condition. The definition of epilepsy requires the occurrence of at least one epileptic seizure' and then again in 2014, a further revision was made. Epilepsy was a disease of the brain defined by any of the following conditions: (i) at least two unprovoked (or reflex) seizures occurring more than 24 hours apart; (ii) one unprovoked (or reflex) seizure and a probability of further seizures similar to the general recurrence risk (at least 60%) after two unprovoked seizures, occurring over the next 10 years; (iii) diagnosis of an epilepsy syndrome. The latest definition is the first to call epilepsy a disease, seemingly oblivious of the difficulties of this concept, and both the 2006 and 2014 definitions get tangled up in the question of seizure-recurrence or seizure-number both of which in reality should be a footnote, not a feature, of the main definition. This seems to us to have strayed far too far from the essential nature of a condition and to tarry around its periphery. The 2006 definition is notable for acknowledging the fact that having epilepsy is more than having seizures but this was again ignored in 2014. The merry-go-round goes around, but Jackson's fundamental definition remains at its still centre.

International League Against Epilepsy Classifications

Classification, like definition, is important for communication and precision in clinical practice, and also provides a framework through which to conceptualise knowledge and research. A badly formulated scheme risks futile or unfocused research and it is therefore a topic of great significance. Jackson himself was very exercised by the question of classification in epilepsy, and what he wrote still stands today. He distinguished between what he called a scientific classification and one that he considered 'purely utilitarian'. He used the analogy of a classification of plants. The scientific classification was based on taxonomy and is what a botanist might use, by providing a listing of natural classes, for instance of species, genera, phyla, and so on. The utilitarian classification, on the other hand, is what a gardener might use and is 'such an arrangement [that] goes by what is most superficial or striking' (for instance, the colour, the size, or the time of flowering). Jackson pointed out that the gardener's classification, useful for day-to-day purposes, is not 'a natural classification. However much of it may be further elaborated, it makes not even an approach to a scientific classification.' A distinction needs to be made between classifications of epileptic seizures and classifications of epilepsy, although in the many proposals made over the years, this distinction has been sometimes mixed up. Some classification schemes are more physiologically based and some more clinical and others more sociological. The most influential have been those of the ILAE.

The starting point of the foray of the ILAE into classification was the seizures type classification. In 1964 and again in 1969, Henry Gastaut,[13] who was then ILAE President, convened meetings to produce an 'ILAE classification of seizure type' (i.e. a classification of epileptic seizures) (Figures 1.5 and 1.6). Gastaut was a brilliant, energetic but autocratic person, and the process he initiated was mired in controversy and disagreement, but in 1969, a version which he had personally largely created and promoted, was published and became widely adopted. Seizures were described mainly according to their clinical form but also their EEG appearance (both during seizures and in between seizures) anatomy, aetiology, and age. The main divisions were into 'partial' and 'generalised' seizure types, each further subdivided. Gastaut was careful not to use the term 'focal' to refer to 'partial' seizures as he realised that a network involving sometimes wide areas of cortex underpinned many partial seizures. This distinction, despite Gastaut's emphasis, has now regrettably been lost again in recent ILAE revisions.

The classification was revised in 1981, under the leadership of the ILAE President Fritz Dreifuss,[14] who like Gastaut was another towering figure in the history of epilepsy. Anatomy, age, and aetiology were removed as criteria because 'they were largely based on historical or speculative information rather than information based on direct observation'. The 1981 classification became therefore an 'electro-clinical classification' restricted entirely to clinical and EEG data and was a true gardener's classification. It became widely adopted and has become the lingua franca of epilepsy specialists around the world to this day. In our opinion, from the medical perspective, this still remains the most useful, at least for practical medical purposes, classification to use.

Much less successful was the ILAE's attempt to produce a classification of the epilepsies in addition to the seizure type classification. This was first drafted in 1985 and approved by the ILAE in 1989, in parallel to the classification of epileptic seizures. One reason for its lack of success was the decision, mistaken

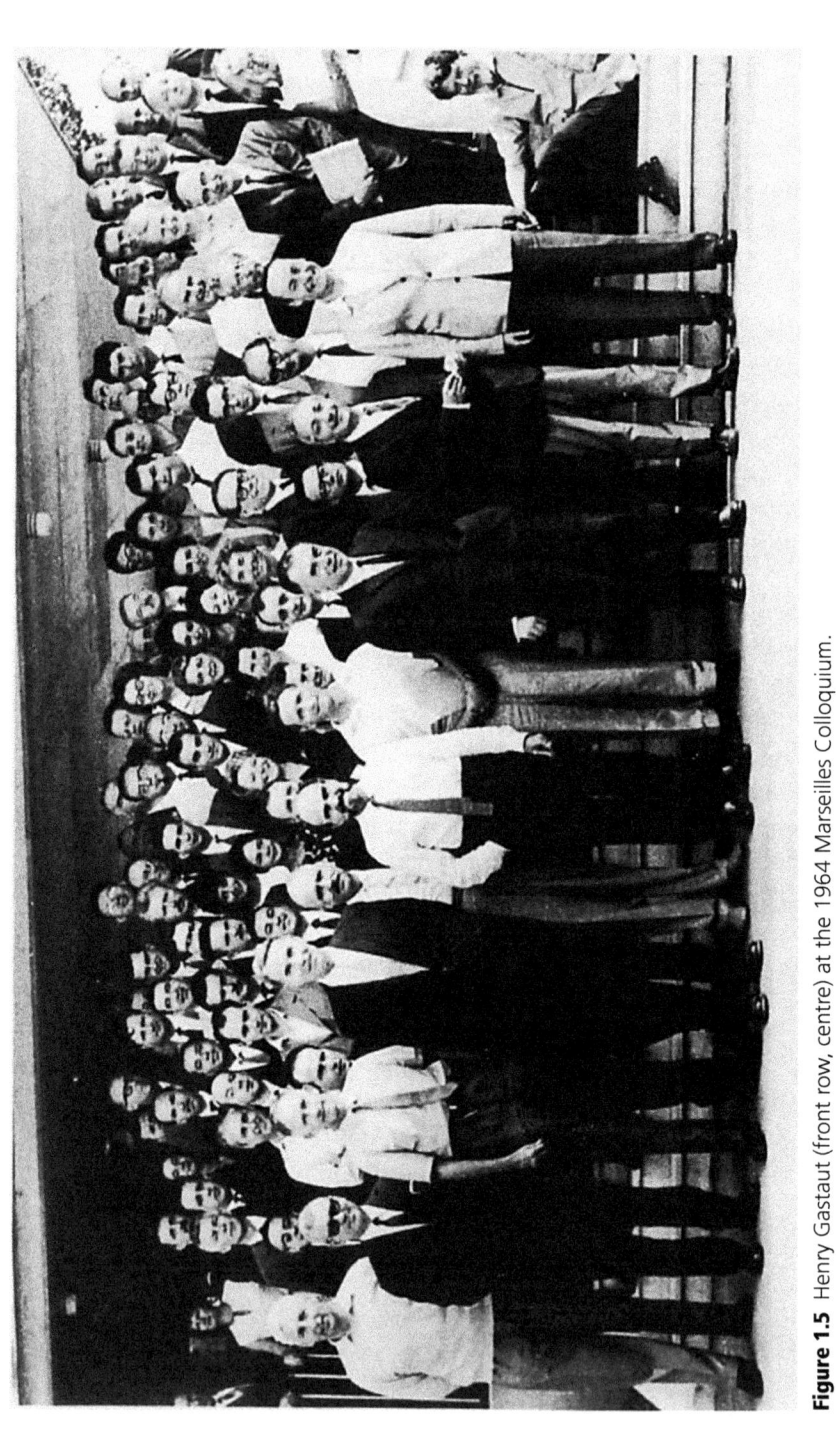

Figure 1.5 Henry Gastaut (front row, centre) at the 1964 Marseilles Colloquium. Reproduced with permission from Dravet C and Roger J. In Memoriam: Henri Gastaut 1915–1995. *Epilepsia*, Volume 37, Issue 4, pp. 410–415, Copyright © 1996 John Wiley and Sons.

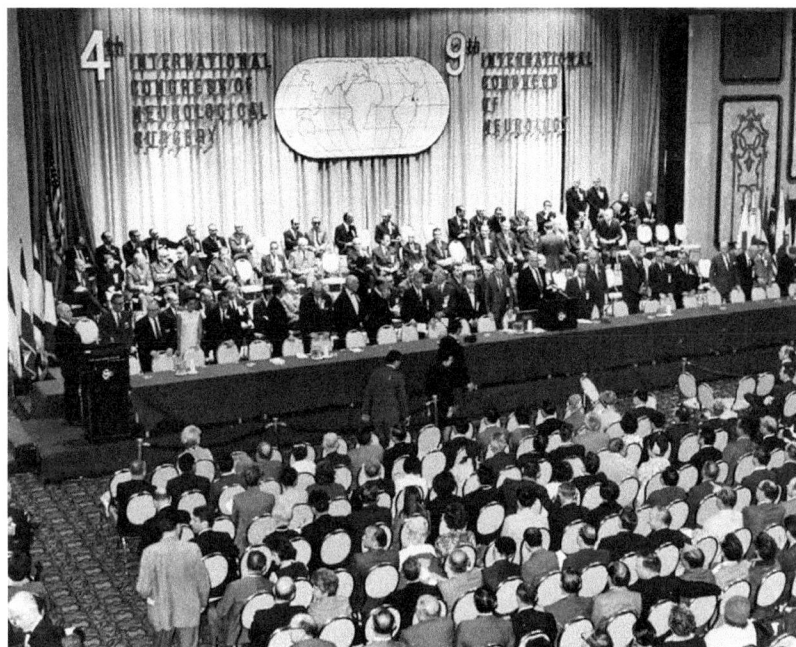

Figure 1.6 The International Congress of Neurology held in the Hilton Hotel in New York in 1969 at which the 11th International Congress of the ILAE was held at 27 September 1969. The celebrated 1969 Classification of Epileptic Seizure Type was debated at this meeting.
Reproduced by kind permission of World Federation of Neurosurgical Societies, Switzerland. Copyright © 2016 World Federation of Neurosurgical Societies.

in our view, to divide epilepsy into generalised and partial types, as already had been done for seizures. This proved a recipe for confusion, and inevitable havoc was the result as seizures and epilepsy began to be used interchangeably. The second reason was to largely ignore aetiology, which was after all one of main justifications for calling 'epilepsy' a 'disease'. Furthermore, the classification completely ignored the broader significance of the term epilepsy, and was, in our view, a lost opportunity.

In 1997, the ILAE set up a new Task Force on Classification and Terminology which produced a succinct glossary of terms (referred to earlier) in 2001, and in the same year a paper on classification, proposing a diagnostic scheme and the idea of breaking up the unitary classification into several 'listings' using different axes—for example, seizure type, syndrome, aetiology, and impairment. This idea was borrowed from similar work in psychiatry and is useful for clinical practice, even if not providing a synoptical framework for classification. Wisely the Task Force declared that it was not possible at this time to produce a new classification scheme. However, the term 'diagnostic scheme' was confusing and the process was soon widely believed to be an attempt at classification. In 2006 and 2010, more listings were made and the Task Force also suggested changes in terminology. This latter development was not only unnecessary and inaccurate, but has sown the seeds for immense confusion in the wider medical and lay communities. As we write, epilepsy classification, which has always been difficult and contentious, is now in a greater state of chaos than at any time in the last 50 years. What is really needed is a 'botanical' classification, one entrenched in the new insights of physiology and molecular science—perhaps dividing the epilepsies into neurochemical syndromes or networks or systems. It is perhaps obvious that we are not ready for this as yet, but work should be directed towards it. Then a new classification would make sense, which is more than just changing terminology or making minor changes around the edge of old systems.

The Current Position

So where are we now? It is clear that there are difficulties in defining epilepsy, of assigning 'disease' status to it, and that what it signifies depends on the perspective taken. The medical and social perspectives come up with very different perceptions of the condition. Some will take the view that this is dancing on the head of a pin, and that 'we know a disease when we see one'. But this is an illusion. Cultural, social, and other considerations greatly affect how we consider a condition like epilepsy, and the lack of any satisfactory definition is evidence of this. The concept of epilepsy has also changed historically, and it is the arrogance of youth to consider now always superior to the past.

To be able to categorise a condition though, is important for all sorts of financial, legal, societal, psychological, as well as medical purposes and for this reason, a definition is needed. There are important differences also between disability and disease, and the experience of epilepsy as disability may differ markedly from the experience of epilepsy as a medical condition—issues of personal identity, social reactions, and individual rights can take centre stage. When it comes to 'seizures'—the 'symptom' of 'epilepsy'—the medical perspective is less challenged, and there is a clear physiological basis which firmly anchors definition. However, even so, there are a penumbra of electrographic and clinical phenomena which may or may not be classed as seizures.

If definition has run into difficulties, classification is in an even greater mess. This is an area where, if useful changes are to be made, the classifiers need to go back to basics. What we all seek is a botanical classification, not a gardener's classification. A classification of seizures should reflect the inherent nature of the seizure—its physiological and chemical systems nature—and not simply its outward appearance. The distinction between tonic–clonic, absence, and partial seizures is surely exactly the same as the distinction between red, yellow, and white roses in the gardener's classification of a rose. We surely can do better than this. When it comes to classifying epilepsy (in contrast to seizures) the problem is much greater. We can in part retreat to Lennox's position and agree that this is fundamentally dependant on 'cause' but then run into difficulties about assigning cause. When wider social, commercial, economic, political, personal, and psychological aspects are added to the mix, classification becomes even more complex. Changing terminology, which has been one aspect of current attempts, is distressingly off the point (in other words, changing the name of an entity without changing its meaning). How to proceed is not clear, and what epilepsy needs is another John Hughlings Jackson to extract us from the very same mire of confusion which he faced at the beginning of our modern era.

Notes

1. No earlier Greek writings have survived. The identity of the author(s) is unknown.
2. In one of his most interesting insights, he equated 'cause' with 'causal mechanism' and was in general not particularly interested in the question of aetiology in the sense usual today; his focus was firmly on theories of physiology. In 1874, he wrote that: 'The confusion of two things physiology and pathology under one (pathology) leads to confusion in considering "causes". Thus, for example, we hear it epigrammatically said that chorea is "only a symptom" and may depend on many causes. This is possibly true of pathological causation; in other words it may be granted that various abnormal nutritive processes may lead to that functional change in grey matter which, when established, admits occasional excessive discharge. But physiologically, that is to say, from the point of view of Function, there is but one cause of chorea—viz. instability of nerve tissue. Similarly in any epilepsy, there is but "one cause" physiologically speaking—viz. the instability of the grey matter, but an unknown number of causes if we mean pathological processes leading to that instability'.
3. Jean-Martin Charcot (1825–1893), a renowned French neurologist, was one of the founders of modern neurology. He had a special interest in epilepsy and in particular in hysterical seizures.
4. These are beyond the scope of this book, but readers are referred to the standard texts on the neurophysiology of epilepsy for further information.
5. William Gordon Lennox (1884–1960) was the leading American epilepsy specialist of his time. He was a leading researcher on EEG, at a time when it was first introduced, and a historian of epilepsy. He set up and directed the famous Epilepsy Unit in Boston, Massachusetts, and worked as Professor of Neurology at Harvard Medical School and was President of the International League Against Epilepsy from 1935 to 1943. He, with his wife, wrote a standard monograph on epilepsy (6).
6. For the authors' view and further discussion on these points, see Shorvon (7,8).
7. See Bashfield (9) for a discussion of the historical evolution of psychiatric thought.
8. For a further discussion of this, and the views of the authors on this issue, see Johnson and Shorvon (11).

9. William Bateson (1861–1926) coined the word genetics, and was a key thinker in the early history of modern genetics. His phrase 'Treasure your exceptions' derives from his inaugural lecture at the University of Cambridge in 1908 (12) and is the title of an important biography of Bateson (13).
10. Scully is Professor of Social Ethics and Bioethics at the University of Newcastle, United Kingdom.
11. Various neuropathologists and neurologists, whose names have been eponymously associated with pathological conditions, based their experiments on brain tissue from those killed in concentration camps. These included Julius Hallervorden, who studied 697 brains from victims of euthanasia in concentration camps and it is alleged that he was present at the killing of more than 60 children and removed the brains himself, and also Hugo Spatz, Friedrich Wegener, and Hans Joachim Scherer.
12. For a description of the evolution of ILAE definitions and classifications of epilepsy and epileptic seizures, and details of the authors' appraisal, see Shorvon (15).
13. Henri Jean Pascal Gastaut (1915–1995) was a French neurologist and the leading theoretician on epilepsy of his period. He held many positions, including the Deanship of the University of Marseille School of Medicine and served on the ILAE executive committee between 1953 and 1977. He made major contributions in many areas of epilepsy, including masterminding the ILAE Classifications of Seizure Type and of the Epilepsies.
14. Fritz E. Dreifuss (1926–1997) was a German-born American neurologist, educated in New Zealand, trained in England, and who became the leading American epilepsy specialist of his time. He worked as Professor of Neurology in Charlottesville, Virginia, where he built up a renowned epilepsy unit. He trained many future leaders and made many clinical and research contributions, especially in the field of classification. He pioneered the establishment of the Comprehensive Epilepsy Programs in the United States. He served as ILAE President between 1985 and 1989 and led the organisation at a period of great expansion.

References

1. **Temkin O.** *The Falling Sickness: A History of Epilepsy from the Greeks to the Beginnings of Modern Neurology.* Baltimore, MD: Johns Hopkins University Press; 1945.
2. **Shorvon SD.** The evolution of epilepsy theory and practice at the National Hospital for the Relief and Cure of Epilepsy, Queen Square between 1860 and 1910. *Epilepsy Behav* 2014; **31**:228–242.
3. **Jackson JH.** A study of convulsions. *Trans St Andrews Med Grad Assoc* 1869, 1870; **3**:162–204.
4. **Jackson JH.** On the anatomical, physiological, and pathological investigations of epilepsies. *West Riding Lunatic Asylum Med Rep* 1873, **3**:315–349.
5. **Elliott B, Joyce E, Shorvon S.** Delusions, illusions and hallucinations in epilepsy: 2. Complex phenomena and psychosis. *Epilepsy Res* 2009; **85**:172–186.
6. **Lennox W, Lennox M.** *Epilepsy and Related Disorders.* Boston, MA: Little Brown; 1960.
7. **Shorvon S.** The concept of symptomatic epilepsy and the complexities of assigning cause in epilepsy. *Epilepsy Behav* 2014; **32**:1–8.

8. **Shorvon S.** Historical introduction: the causes of epilepsy in the pre-molecular era (1860–1960). In: Shorvon SD, Andermann F, Guerrini R (eds) *The Causes of Epilepsy: Common and Uncommon Causes in Adults and Children.* Cambridge: Cambridge University Press; 2011:1–20.
9. **Bashfield RK.** *The Classification of Psychopathology.* New York: Plenum Press; 1984.
10. **Illich I.** *Limits to Medicine.* London: Marion Boyars; 1976.
11. **Johnson MR, Shorvon SD.** Heredity in epilepsy: neurodevelopment, comorbidity, and the neurological trait. *Epilepsy Behav* 2011; **22**:421–427.
12. **Bateson W.** *The Methods and Scope of Genetics: An Inaugural Lecture Delivered 23 October 1908.* Cambridge: Cambridge University Press; 1908.
13. **Cock A, Forsdyke DR.** *Treasure Your Exceptions: The Science and Life of William Bateson.* New York: Springer; 2008.
14. **Scully JL.** What is a disease? *EMBO Rep* 2004; **5**(7):650–653.
15. **Shorvon S.** Definition (terminology) and classification in epilepsy: a historical survey and current formulation, with special reference to the ILAE. In: Shorvon S, Perucca E, Engel J (eds) *Treatment of Epilepsy.* Oxford: Wiley; 2015:1–23.

Chapter 2
Attitudes

'What has been the most important improvement in the treatment of epilepsy in the modern era?' This question is at the heart of our book. Was it the discovery of new antiepileptic drugs (AEDs), the introduction of EEG or magnetic resonance imaging (MRI), or the surgery of the brain? In our view, perhaps surprisingly, the answer lies in none of these, important as they are. Each is entrenched in the medical model of the disease and each overemphasises the doctors' perspective. Epilepsy is not only, or even most importantly, just a medical condition, but it is also something that happens to people, and that may ruin lives and livelihoods. Let's not forget that many people with epilepsy have a few seizures and are at no social disadvantage, but have suffered terribly from societal attitudes, and some still do. It is the history of these attitudes and the recent improvements that are the topic of this chapter.

It is our view that it is the change in attitudes of society and medicine towards people with epilepsy, and the changes in the way that society has dealt with epilepsy in the past 30 years, above all else, that has had the greatest impact on the lives of sufferers. In the first hundred years of our modern era, being 'epileptic' was a nightmare of prejudice and stigma, and, as we shall relate, on occasions resulted even in violence against the person or death. Seismic social changes have occurred and in the past three decades a new understanding of societal responsibilities has formed. This is a success story. Of course not all is rosy, but things are incomparably better than they were at any time in the earlier period.

Society and Epilepsy 1860–1900, and Theories of Degeneration

Before the nineteenth century, many religious and medical authorities considered epilepsy to be a form of possession by the devil, and this was also a general view held by most people in both educated and uneducated strata of the population. Attitudes softened as time had passed, under the impact of the European enlightenment, and as the modern scientific age dawned, this belief was replaced by more scientific concepts.

In the late nineteenth century, though, the fortunes of those with epilepsy had scarcely improved. The first action of the reformers of the mid-nineteenth century was to move the epileptic person out of sight. Asylums had traditionally mixed the insane and the epileptic together, and fettered both, but as the century drew on, there was an increasing desire to separate the two, with the intention mainly of protecting the insane from developing epilepsy. Initially, epileptic wards were set up in most lunatic asylums but towards the end of the century, separate institutions specifically for people with epilepsy began to be created in Europe and the United States; examples were the centres at Bethel in Germany, Chalfont in the United Kingdom, and Blackwell's Island (now Roosevelt Island) in the United States. These were often established with good intentions by philanthropists, but their actions were the consequence of the predominant societal view of the time that the person with epilepsy was someone not suitable for mixing in polite society, and who should be excluded as much as possible despite the fact that the slur of demonic possession was no longer widely arrogated. These policies of exclusion permeated all aspects of life, including marriage, employment, and education, and the 'epileptic' was doomed to inhabit the periphery and outer circles of existence.

Sieveking,[1] whose book on epilepsy in 1858 (and the second edition in 1861) was a reflection of advanced beliefs about epilepsy at the dawn of the new scientific age (Figure 2.1), dismisses possession by writing that 'no one contends that there is any form of disease in the present day which is seriously to be attributed to the influences of evil spirits, unless it be the spirit of gin and brandy'! Sieveking did, however, believe that the sight of an epileptic seizure can induce one in the person observing it. He noted too the hereditable influence, and had theories relating to diseases of the bowels and kidneys, but as he pointed out, these were difficult to prove not least as 'epileptics are always desultory patients, it is more difficult to collect their secretions for twenty-four hours'. It was though the relationship of epilepsy to the 'sexual organs' which attracted special attention in Sieveking's view. He believed that masturbation commonly induced epilepsy by 'enfeebling' the system. As he wrote:

> Amongst the twenty-nine male epileptics of my second analysis of fifty-two cases, I find no less than nine in whom the sexual system was in a state of great excitement, owning to recent or former masturbation ... In a person guilty of masturbation, we generally notice a peculiar hang-dog expression; an unwillingness to meet the speaker eye to eye; a large sluggish pupil; a pale livid hue and languid circulation of the surface, a general nervousness of demeanour.

The idea that epilepsy was caused by self-masturbation was one that was widely accepted until the middle years of the twentieth century.

Another major preoccupation of European society in the late nineteenth century was the perception that civilised society was degenerating, due to the rise of urban poor, and this engaged the anxieties of anthropologists, sociologists,

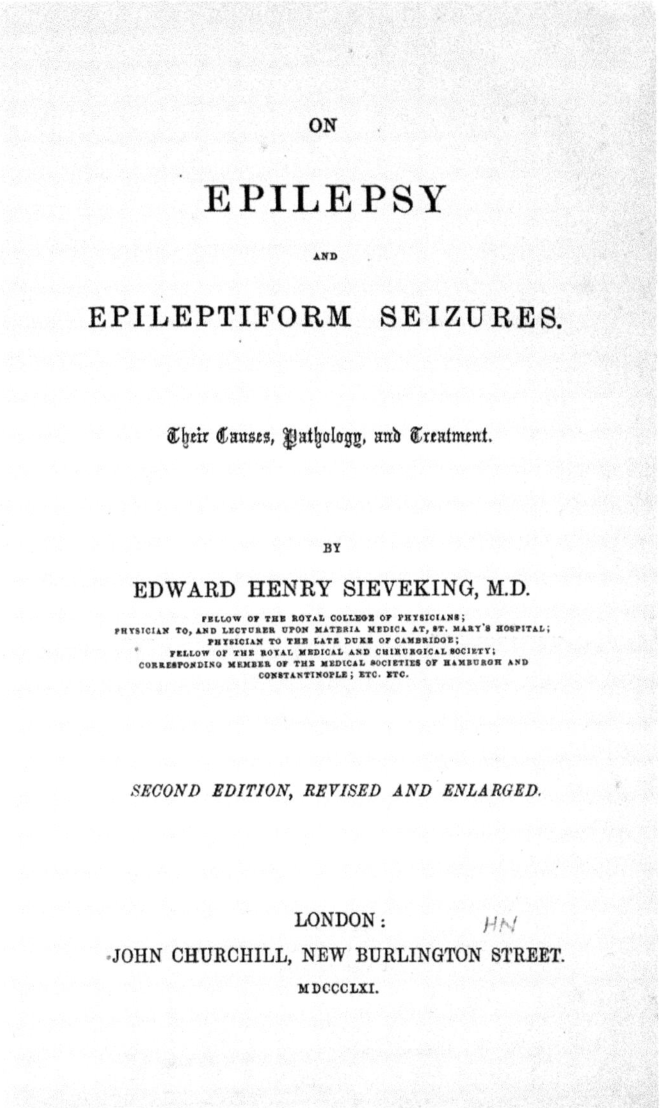
ON

EPILEPSY

AND

EPILEPTIFORM SEIZURES.

Their Causes, Pathology, and Treatment.

BY

EDWARD HENRY SIEVEKING, M.D.

FELLOW OF THE ROYAL COLLEGE OF PHYSICIANS;
PHYSICIAN TO, AND LECTURER UPON MATERIA MEDICA AT, ST. MARY'S HOSPITAL;
PHYSICIAN TO THE LATE DUKE OF CAMBRIDGE;
FELLOW OF THE ROYAL MEDICAL AND CHIRURGICAL SOCIETY;
CORRESPONDING MEMBER OF THE MEDICAL SOCIETIES OF HAMBURGH AND CONSTANTINOPLE; ETC. ETC.

SECOND EDITION, REVISED AND ENLARGED.

LONDON:
JOHN CHURCHILL, NEW BURLINGTON STREET.
MDCCCLXI.

Figure 2.1 Title page of Sir Edward Sieveking's celebrated book on epilepsy which opens the modern era, the second edition was published in 1861.

novelists, politicians, and social commentators as well as doctors. Medical theories mirrored social attitudes and the theories of mental degeneration were developed to their fullest extent by the French psychiatrist Bénédict Augustin Morel who took the view that the genetic stock of the population was degenerating, and there was in particular a group of inherited conditions which resulted in a *progressive* deterioration (degeneration) of the physical, mental, and moral fibre of the afflicted individual.[2] Epilepsy was at the centre of this group of conditions, inherited together as what was known as the 'Neurological Trait', which also included insanity, dementia, mental retardation, general paralysis, and sometimes moral degeneracy.[3] The concept of inherited degeneracy struck a chord with the general public, and this fin de siècle preoccupation with spiritual decomposition discerned a ready example in the person with epilepsy who found himself or herself right at the centre of this maelstrom. The importance of the theories of degeneration for patients with epilepsy in this period cannot be overestimated in terms of the stigmatisation they caused and the negative stereotypes of epilepsy which became almost universally held. There were very few neurologists or psychiatrists of that period who did not accept Morel's concept.

Another negative strand of the concept of the neuropathic trait, also universally held up to the mid-twentieth century, was the perception that people with epilepsy had disturbed mental states and a characteristic (epileptic) personality. Morel believed that the suffering of a person with epilepsy led to increasing irritability which resulted in a 'perversion in their ideas and feelings'. Kraepelin emphasised aggressiveness. Viscosity or an adhesive personality was noted by many, who attached to the epileptic patient such terminology as enechetic constitution, ixoid character, or glischroid type. Turner could write in 1907 (3), 'It is rare to find epileptics who do not present some form of mental obliquity' and viewed this as a sign of their 'hereditarily degenerative disposition'. He believed epileptics to be 'on the whole self-opinionated and egotistical, and possess a conceit and assurance which is out of all proportion to their achievements; their conversations are usually prolix and pretentious. In character they are mobile and unstable'. Turner found them often tenacious, possessing religious fervour (a marked feature of their disease) and which contrasted strongly with their actions 'which are often perverted, passionate and immoral. Their ideas of right and wrong are often vague'. In the United States, Leon Pierce Clark (4) found: 'The child who is to be an epileptic is vicious, already irritable and impulsive, His motives are futile, he isolates himself or runs away, and has sombre ideas. At the slightest reprimand he speaks of suicide, or absents himself for days after a chiding. He is sexually precocious, an onanist, has night terrors, somnambulism etc'. This may seem extraordinary language from a leading American epilepsy specialist, but surely reflects the attitudes then prevalent and also the lack of constraint in expressing them. Clark wrote further that the epileptic suffers from a temperamental defect, a personality defect which makes social adaptation impossible, the sufferer regressing to a state of 'metroerotism' (uterine fantasy). Clark continues: 'there is a more or less constant affective defect in all epileptics, sane as well as insane; that such defect is due to an inherent make-up of the psyche in which mainly an egocentricity and a highly sensitized feeling are given to the individual'. He will intellectually as well as emotionally gradually degenerate into the so-called epileptic dementia.

The perceived personality faults of epileptics, and association with psychiatric disorder and feeblemindedness, linked with the theories of degeneration, were a toxic mixture; and perhaps inevitably a new 'scientific' theory became the oxygen that ignited these smouldering fires. Social Darwinism, an umbrella name for this new scientific trend which had many manifestations, sought to provide a biological explanation for social phenomenon. An important early example was that of the work of Lombroso[4] who devised the notion that criminality was linked to epilepsy, and indeed that 'great criminality was a form of equivalence of epilepsy' (Table 2.1). He noted, by impressive

Table 2.1 Anomalies shared by epileptics and criminals as published by Cesare Lombroso

Anatomical feature	Features considered by Lombroso to be shared by epileptics and criminals
Skull	Abnormally large, microcephaly, asymmetric (12–37%), sclerosis, med. occ. fossetta, abnormal indices, large orbital arches, low sloping forehead, wormian bones, simple cranial sutures
Face	Overdeveloped jaw, jutting cheekbones, large jug ears, facial asymmetry, strabismus, virility (in women), anomalous teeth
Brain	Anomalous convolutions, low weight, hypertrophied cerebellum, symptoms of meningitis
Body	Asymmetrical torso, prehensile feet, hernia
Skin	Wrinkles, beardlessness, olive skin, tattoos, delayed grey hair/balding, dark and curly hair
Motor anomalies	Left handedness (10%), abnormal reflexes, heightened agility (16%)
Sensory anomalies	Tactile insensitivity (81%), insensitivity to pain, overly acute eyesight, dullness of hearing, taste and smell
Psychological anomalies (% in epileptics)	Limited intelligence (30–69%), weak memory (14–91%), Hallucinations (20–41%), superstitious, blunted emotions, love of animals, absence of remorse, impulsivity (2–50%), cannibalism and ferocity, pederasty (2–39%), masturbation (21–67%), perversity (15–57%), vanity, sloth, passion for gaming, mania/paranoia, delirium, dizziness, delusions of grandeur (1–3%), irascibility (30–100%), lying (7–100%), theft (4–75%), religious delusions (14–100%)
Causes	Heredity (of alcoholism, insanity, epilepsy, old parents), alcoholism

Source: data from Lombroso C. *L'uomo delinquent*, Fourth Edition. Milan: Hoepli, 1876; and Lombroso C. *L'uomo delinquent*, Fifth Edition. Milan: Hoepli, 1896.

leaps of mental acrobatics, similarities in the physiognomy of criminals and of epileptics. He drew the conclusion that epilepsy and crime (and bizarrely genius) had a common pathogenesis, namely a defect in the development of the central nervous system which resulted in deficient ethics and behaviour. Lombroso's ideas evolved over time, and in their fully developed form he held that two-thirds of criminal individuals were 'born criminals' who inherited a criminal trait and possessed 'anomalies' (physical and psychological) resembling the traits of primitive man and animals (and even plants) (Figure 2.2). These traits were *atavistic throwbacks* to a primitive stage in human evolution, and he considered epilepsy to be one such atavistic characteristic and a fundamental component of the criminal type. He produced lists of characteristics shared by criminals and epileptics and observed that 26.9% of all epileptic men and 25% of all epileptic women have a 'full criminal type' from the physiognomic point of view. He furthermore, following similar theories of Morel and others, suggested that some criminals exhibited 'hidden epilepsy' (epilessia larvata) manifest by 'sharp, sudden outbursts … the psychological equivalents of physical seizures, marked by unpredictability and ferocity': and that this hidden epilepsy was responsible for criminal acts, especially acts of physical or sexual violence. This theory, like the parallel theories of the neuropathic trait and of degeneration, was widely accepted. It, too, entered public discourse, and found its way into the arts of the time, and a classic example of hidden epilepsy and the epileptic type is to be found in the character and crimes of Roubaud and Lantier in Zola's *La bête Humaine* (Figure 2.3). Lennox (5) noted that Lombroso's experiences were based on his examination of bromide-soaked, feeble-minded institutionalised cases, and this may be a partial explanation, but the perception of a close association between crime and epilepsy is retained by some to this day.

The Twentieth Century: The Descent and Rise of Societal Attitudes

Thus, in the first years of the twentieth century, the public perception of epileptic people was at a low point. Tarred by the brush of masturbation, degeneration, personality disturbance, idiocy, and criminality, it is not surprising that strenuous efforts were made by many individuals and families to hide the symptoms of epilepsy. The person with epilepsy kept the fact well under wraps and if the seizures were frequent was often sheltered from the public gaze. A classic case is that of Prince John, the fifth son of Britain's King George V, born in 1905 and who developed epilepsy at the age of 4 years, and died in a seizure at the age of 18 years. He was hidden away in the Sandringham estate, beloved by his mother

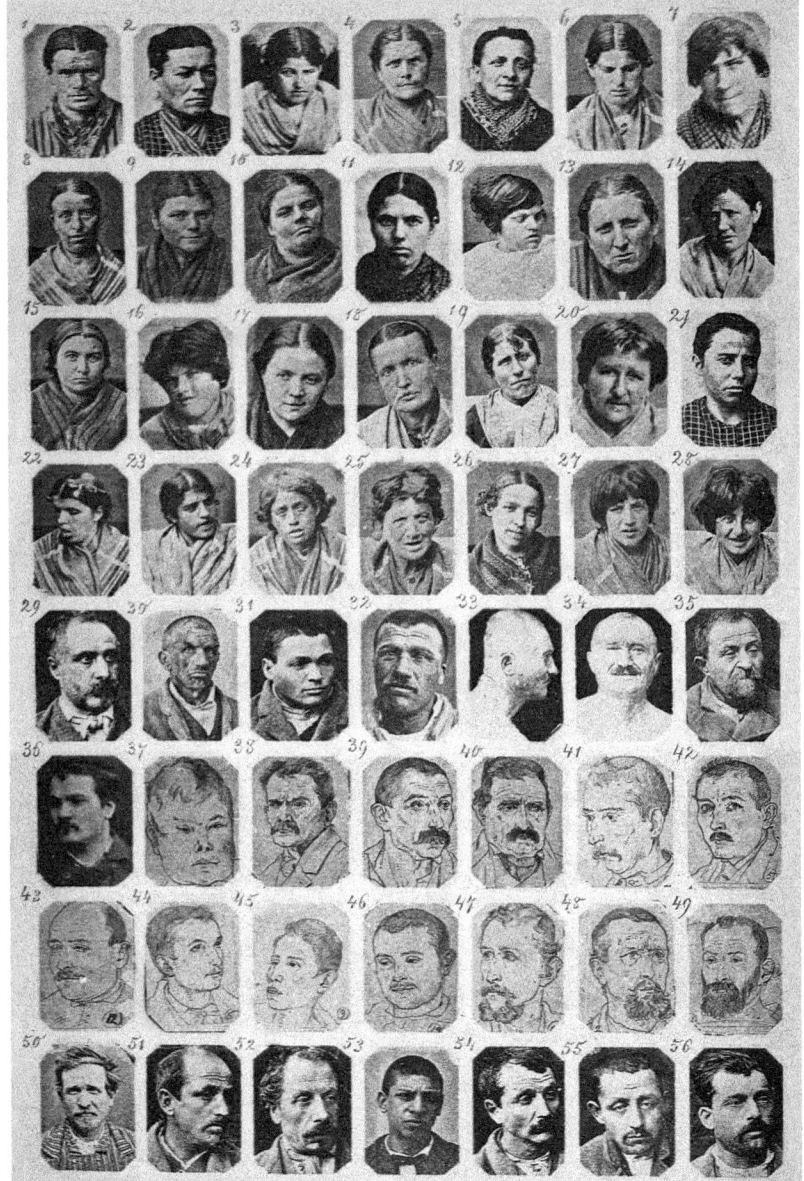

Figure 2.2 An illustration from *L'uomo delinquente* by Cesare Lombroso, purporting to show the physiognomy of epilepsy.
Reproduced from Lombroso C. *L'uomo delinquente*, Milan: Hoepli, 1876.

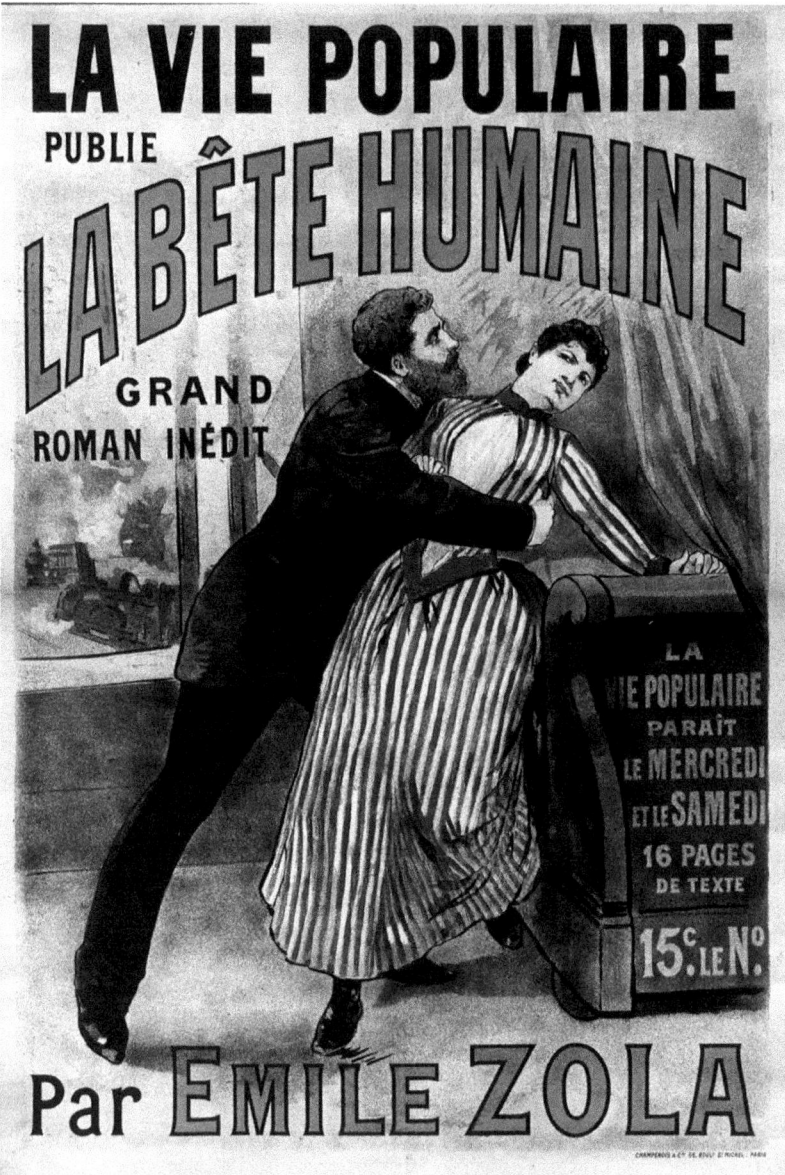

Figure 2.3 Reproduced by kind permission of the Bibliothèque nationale de France. Copyright © 2016 Bibliothèque nationale de France.

but considered by his brother, the future king Edward VIII, 'more of an animal than anything else'. This attitude, well named the 'canker of secrecy' by Lennox remains to this day in some quarters. It does grievous damage to the individual and one might add to the society whose attitudes engender it.

Scientists, including medical doctors, were largely responsible for providing 'evidence' to back up these, sometimes seemingly bizarre and prejudicial, theories of aetiology of epilepsy, but it should not be forgotten that science itself is moulded by societal attitudes and that the scientists are acting within a social context. Theories reflect the complex interaction of science and society, and not any 'absolute truth' or objectivity, and nothing more strongly illustrates the relativism of science than the rise of social Darwinism and the evolutionary theories of degeneration. It is a mistake to see 'science' as immutable or to have a superior 'truth'. Most of the theories of that time (and indeed today) turn out to be very faulty interpretations of biology.

In the twentieth century, one strand of social Darwinist thinking was to prove a particular tragedy for epileptic people, and this was the theory of eugenics. Eugenics was, for its founder Francis Galton,[5] a method of rational planning of human breeding: the application of 'selection' to human reproduction based on statistical probabilities. His aim was either to encourage the birth of superior lives (positive eugenics) or to prevent the birth of inferior lives (negative eugenics). Its most extreme forms, forcible sterilisation to prevent life or the ultimate step of 'euthanasia' to end lives, were not contemplated by Galton or the first-generation eugenicists, but, appallingly, for epilepsy these became the eventual consequence. In the early twentieth century, the serried ranks of distinguished scientists, doctors, and politicians had replaced the bishops, inquisitors, and cardinals as the major agents of stigma.

The story of eugenics in epilepsy starts in the celebrated scientific research laboratories at Cold Spring Harbor, New York. In 1904, Charles B. Davenport, a leading American scientist and later Professor of Zoology at Harvard University, was appointed Director. To Davenport, a fanatical eugenicist, 'Heredity stands as the one great hope of the human race' and he began to investigate ways of improving the American stock. In 1910, Davenport set up his notorious Eugenics Record Office at Cold Spring Harbor, and began collecting family trees. Epilepsy was a focus of his attention and he published, in 1911, a paper entitled 'A first study of inheritance of epilepsy', co-authored by David Weeks, the superintendent of the Skillman Village for Epileptics which was a hitherto peaceful farm colony in New Jersey set up along the lines of the Bethel Colony in Germany, and who was later appointed to the executive of the ILAE (6). It is a horrifying study of 175 family trees of inmates in the Colony. The authors' intent is clear from the beginning and highly inaccurate descriptions of the families are given, following this sort of standard pattern:

> The central mating is between an epileptic women (descended from an epileptic mother) and a sot, whose mother was insane and who is himself sexually immoral and infected both with gonorrhea and syphilis. The first child is epileptic, the next two are

neurotic, No. 3 has hysteria and No. 4 died in infancy. There followed thirteen miscarriages, clearly due to the infection.

Davenport and Weeks conclude that the epilepsy is a manifestation of the neuropathic taint, which results in the lack of 'some element necessary for complete mental development'. They then went on to predict that, given the mating patterns and fecundity, that there will be an exponential increase in the population numbers of epileptic and feeble minded people in the community of New Jersey unless urgent measures are taken. They concluded that 'segregation during the entire reproductive period violates least the social ideals of our time' but later that sterilisation of the unfit was the one method which could most effectively 'dry up the springs that feed the torrent of defective and degenerative protoplasm'. Both Weeks and Davenport gave public speeches and gave expert evidence to legislative and public bodies, and there was soon public pressure to pass laws first to prevent marriage of epileptics and then to allow their enforced sterilisation. By 1914, people with epilepsy were specifically prohibited from marriage in 13 States of the United States. Davenport though felt that compulsory sterilisation was preferable (he actually preferred castration to vasectomy, as he considered that it also reduced lust) and the pressure to legislate about this also grew. The legal case of *Buck* v. *Bell* was a landmark in this history. These infamous proceedings, heard first in Virginia, took place in the United States Supreme Court where in 1927 Judge Wendell Holmes confirmed the legality of sterilisation with the words (6): 'It is better for all the world, if instead of waiting to execute degenerate offspring for crime or to let them starve for their imbecility, society can prevent those who are manifestly unfit from continuing their kind … Three generations of imbeciles are enough.' The first sterilisation statute had been enacted in Indiana in 1907, and after Wendell Holmes' judgment, a deluge of states followed suit.

There were some who tried to restrain this increasingly violent trend, and there was debate about the ethics and the validity of the science. Nevertheless, the science of eugenics, and the excesses of its ardent practitioners, had caught the public imagination (like much genetics today) and the voices of moderation on behalf of epilepsy were largely drowned out. What was missing, intriguingly, was any well-publicised critique by the patients themselves, and it seems most simply kept their heads down.

An important thing to emphasise was the eugenic movement was based on apparently scientific principles; these provided its legitimacy. The science was flawed, as indeed much science was, and is, largely because the experiments were manipulated sometimes deliberately (and both Goddard and Davenport have been accused of this), but sometimes by the enthusiasm of the scientist keen to get the result that he or she desires. Bias can be introduced in the selection of subjects to study, measurement techniques can be faulty, the scientific question can be poorly drafted, and the statistics misused. In the social sciences and in medicine, it is only too easy to fall into these traps. Indeed, throughout its history, medical science, and especially in relation to disorders of the brain, has been subject to fashion and fancy, with huge effort and large cost expended on fashionable theories that are inherently mistaken and that lead nowhere. Eugenics, psychoanalysis, and many forms of contemporary neuroscience are examples of this.[6]

Eugenics became a worldwide phenomenon and it was in Germany of course that the eugenic theories reached their most extreme form, under the title of racial hygiene. This was seen as both a science and a social movement, and had strong political and legal support. In 1933, the first racial hygiene law was passed for the 'Prevention of hereditarily diseased progeny'. The law sanctioned the compulsory sterilisation by surgery or by X-rays of people suffering from inherited epilepsy. Hereditary Courts were set up which between 1933 and 1949 which sanctioned the sterilisation of 320 000–350 000 people, and in 1935 the law was amended to include eugenic abortion up to the sixth month of pregnancy. The Nazi propaganda machine produced films showing a nation menaced by hordes of feeble-minded people, the cost of caring for whom could be more usefully spent on housing the racially pure poor (Figure 2.4). It was only a matter of time before more active 'euthanasia' policies were adopted, and the darkest side of epilepsy was revealed in the programme named Action T4 in which patients deemed 'incurably sick' by doctors, or in Hitler's own words were examples of 'life unworthy of life', were provided with 'mercy death in one of six killing centres in Germany'.[7] Once the system was refined, doctors in all hospitals and nursing homes were required to fill in a report form on all patients who had been institutionalised for 5 years or more and who had a specified condition, including epilepsy. There were just two questions relating to epilepsy—was there an abnormal personality, and what was the average seizure frequency? Copies of the reporting forms were dispatched to one of a selection of 'expert physicians' and then to the central office where one of three senior experts (*Obergutachter*) had the final word.[8] If they filled out the empty box on the lower left of the form with a red '+', the patient was killed. If they chose to mark it with a blue '–', the patient would be allowed to live. At first, killings were by lethal injection and then gassing was considered more efficacious. In the most efficient setting, patients were transferred from their institutions to the killing centres in buses named the 'Community Patients Transports Service', operated by teams of SS men wearing white coats, to give a professional appearance. The families and the doctors of patients were not told where the patients were, and they were usually killed within 24 hours of

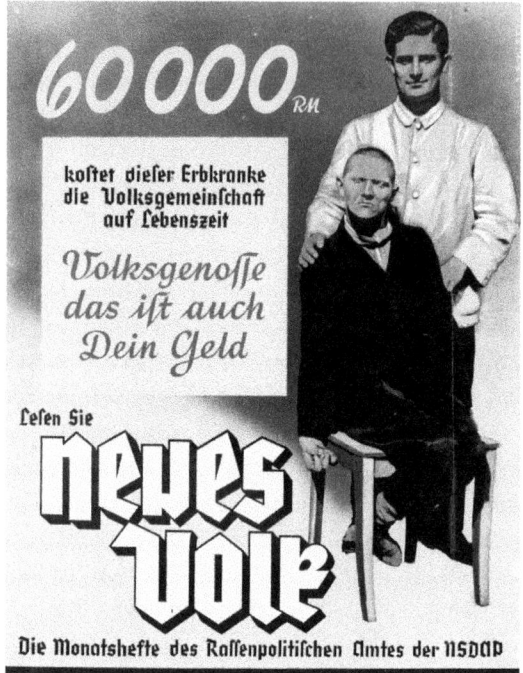

Figure 2.4 Propaganda poster by the Nazi party purporting to show the unacceptable cost of looking after those who were unworthy of life.
Reproduced with permission from the Deutsches Historisches Museum, Berlin. Copyright © 2016 Deutsches Historisches Museum.

leaving. A false but plausible death certificate was sent to the family along with an urn of random ashes. Between 70 000 and 100 000 people were killed in this way, among whom were sometimes perfectly 'sane' epileptics. How many people with epilepsy perished is not known, and when the war was over, eugenicists tried to distance their scientific study from these events but the link was clear. It is worth emphasising that this whole programme was carried out by doctors who colluded with the system, and this cooperation of the medical authorities represents one of the worst transgressions in the history of medicine; nowhere has life been more clearly in breach of universal medical ethical standards or with such subterfuge. Eugenicists were prominent among the doctors prosecuted in the Nuremberg trials, but the usual defence was that the German eugenics differed little from that in the United States, and certainly some escaped punishment on the basis of this argument.

Surprisingly, too, not all were repentant and Racial Hygiene policies, rebranded as Human Genetics, continued in some countries after the war, notably in Switzerland. Prohibition on marriage of people with epilepsy persisted in many countries, and was reiterated, for instance, in the Hindu Marriage act in India of 1955 (and the Special Marriage Act of 1956) which rendered null and void a marriage if one partner was subject to attacks of 'insanity or epilepsy'. In the United States, until 1956, marriage remained barred to people with epilepsy in 17 states, and sterilisation on eugenic grounds was still permitted in 19 states but practised only in 4 according to Lennox (5). Lennox rather innocently reassured us that 'States provide certain safeguards against abuse by means of a eugenic board with physician representation'. The last state to repeal the marriage law did so only in 1980, and in 1960, Lennox reported that even then, eugenic sterilisation was restricted to institutionalised cases only in 13 states, but could be carried out in community-based cases in another 6, and in 11 states laws allowing sterilisation and also prohibiting against marriage was on the statute books. In the United States, it has been estimated that 50 000 sterilisations were carried out. Lennox's opinion was that 'Chief Justice Holmes was wise beyond his time' and that 'eugenics wisely applied can be a force for good … A colony in the South found that sterilisation was directly advantageous to patients because they could then be released for summer work on farms in other parts of the state without fear of undesirable sexual complications'.

Attitudes were slow to change. In 1960, Lennox could still write that, whilst most patients with epilepsy should be given full rights in society, personality traits do exist which inhibit this. He wrote in a way which is illuminating from the point of view of advanced US attitudes circa 1960:

> An unreasonable, stubborn, fault finding, selfish, shallow-minded, tiresomely loquacious and reiterative individual … will not be welcomed in any social group. Over zealousness of doctor or social worker in 'placing' such an individual, may spoil the chances for some more acceptable person later on. However, unpleasant and antisocial traits can often be ameliorated or removed by control of seizures.

Thus, was the opinion of the leading epilepsy specialist in the United States in 1960. To the eminent German psychiatrist Bleuler in 1955, epileptics were found to have, and their relatives also, greater degrees than normal of vagabondage, begging, personal neglect, prostitution, and criminality, have severely slowed trains of thought and sluggishness, and thought which had something unclear and vague about it. Epileptics were wearying, he felt, because of their prolixity, stickiness, perseveration, and emphasis on small and inessential details,

In the face of such prejudice, most people in the community with epilepsy concealed their condition, not surprisingly in view of these stigmatising pronouncements from eminent medical authorities. This made the prejudice worse, as the medical and societal view of the 'epileptic' was strongly coloured by the seeming association of epilepsy with mental retardation and feeblemindedness.

Nevertheless, the strident language and violence which people with epilepsy faced in the first half of the twentieth century was slowly largely quelled in most countries in the next few decades. The shameful events of the war tempered the language and the stigma of epilepsy and since then, an approach began to be taken which was more mindful of human rights. It is interesting to speculate on the reasons. It was not only the uncovering of the wartime extremes such as Action T4 which shamed the public. Perhaps the dignity and lack of complaint in the face of the accumulating stigma was another aspect of the changing relationship. In many places, people with epilepsy were, in the latter part of the twentieth century, more able to come out into the open and were treated more kindly.

Legislation has also helped, including the post-war consensus on human rights, and in every Western country at least there is now strong anti-discrimination legislation. In the United States, for instance, the first law to prohibit discrimination against people with physical disabilities was passed in 1973, but had limited scope and it was only in 1990 that the Americans with Disabilities Act provided real teeth. Until the 1970s, for instance, it was still legal in the United States to deny people with seizures entry to restaurants, theatres, recreational centres, and other public places, but now such restrictions would be entirely socially unacceptable.

Ironically, it was only when this more humanitarian approach developed, that the first studies of stigma in epilepsy were carried out. These show that there remain, despite the disappearance of eugenics, multiple impacts on the lives of patients, and it seems particularly the case in poorer countries. Stigma, as a topic of study, was popularised by Irving Goffman (9). He set the agenda and sociologists since have made much of his important distinction between 'enacted stigma' and 'felt stigma'. Even as society legislates against the former, the latter may linger and people with epilepsy continue to experience both. Research shows adverse effects of the condition on employment, marriage, education, and domestic and family life. It seems that there is a tendency among all people to stigmatise, and although this can be diminished by social or cultural mores, it remains a basic human instinct. The occurrence of seizures tends to frighten onlookers, who do not understand what they are witnessing, and fear translates into a desire to exclude. The US Supreme Court recognised this in 1987 when it ruled that 'a review of the history of epilepsy provides a salient example that fear, rather than the handicap itself, is the major impetus for discrimination against people with handicaps'. Furthermore, the association of epilepsy with mental handicap and psychological disturbance adds the stigma of these conditions to epilepsy.

Stigma casts a long shadow over many aspects of the life of a person with epilepsy, and this in turn leads to a tendency to withdraw from social contact, to feel shame and anticipate rejection, a vulnerability to mental disorder, and engenders sadness and bitterness. One reaction to this by sufferers is to adopt a defensive attitude which itself becomes self-defeating and stigmatising. Prejudice and discrimination become accepted as a routine part of life. Cultural aspects and family support are essential. A recent study looking at the lives of people with epilepsy in Saudi Arabia came to the conclusion that, in this socially conservative country, felt stigma was not very prominent and this was put down to the strongly held religious convictions and strong family support were perceived as core to the person's quality of life (10). Europe, chastened by the experience of the war, has led in legislation to protect people with epilepsy (among other groups previously ostracised) but in the developing world, discrimination is still rife. The picture though is mixed, and recent studies (11) showed in Germany that 15% of parents would prefer their children not to play with a child with epilepsy. The figure is 72% in Taiwan and China. In Nigeria, 47% of teachers are said to believe children with epilepsy are insane, 32% believe epilepsy is contagious, and 27% prefer them not to play with other children. By 2004, a representative survey of the general public in Britain painted a brighter picture, with 95% of respondents agreeing with the statement that people with epilepsy were as intelligent as anyone else, 95% agreeing that they should be allowed to play with other children, 94% believing that they can be successful as other people in their chosen career, 87% believing they can lead a normal life, and only 22% feeling they had more personality problems (12). The survey authors concluded that the expressed attitudes to epilepsy in this UK sample were generally highly favourable, noted that the public attitude to epilepsy had changed considerably compared to surveys in the 1980s, and that 'the full force of past and contemporary social prejudice and misunderstanding' seemed to be diminishing. The authors suggest that, in the developed world at least, 'the trend now is to value rather than reject human differences and to redefine as normal conditions of being (including health conditions and disabilities) previously viewed as abnormal'. They point out that there is a changing language in the media and in medical circles too about disability (see Chapter 1), but noted that the transformation of epilepsy from the moral to the medical domain, from 'badness' to 'sickness' has almost certainly contributed to its decreasing stigma (interestingly, the reverse is true of other conditions). This is a positive message for people with epilepsy. One other point made was that the loss of control in a seizure created ambiguity in the social interactions of a person with epilepsy, destabilising the social order by being unpredictable and out of control.

A less positive survey was carried out in 2013, albeit of a highly selected group of people with epilepsy from support groups, by a British charity which found that 79% of people with epilepsy considered themselves victims of discrimination, 40% have experienced discrimination or exclusion, and 55% of the adults questioned said that they do not disclose their epilepsy to new people they meet for fear of a negative reaction. A survey of more than 5000 people from highly selected populations of patients from support groups in 15 countries in Europe, found that 51% felt that they were subject to stigma and 18% felt highly stigmatised (13). These two surveys are biased towards patients with multiple problems and severe epilepsy, and were not illustrative of the more typical person with epilepsy. In a more representative survey of 1652 patients in the United Kingdom identified through their primary care physicians as taking AEDs for epilepsy, there was a different picture (14). This was an unselected population and strenuous efforts were taken to ensure that the sample was representative of epilepsy as it appears in the community today: 52% of the cohort had had no seizures in the prior year and a further 8% only one seizure. The cohort was asked about impacts of epilepsy on their lives. Those who were free of seizures, or having only the occasional seizure, reported low levels of impact. In adults, the main negative effect was the restriction on driving. For those with ongoing seizures, though, there were significant impacts on the areas of work, social life, and psychological aspects, and in children on education, psychological aspects, social life, and sport. This survey painted an uneven picture, with many patients free of major impact and with others labouring under the effects of epilepsy, but the key message was that this depended a great deal, perhaps not surprisingly, on whether there were ongoing seizures. The authors concluded that seizure control was key to reducing the impact of the condition—which may sound an obvious message but is certainly one worth emphasising.

So, where are we today? Even as we write this, recent articles in a number of national newspapers celebrating 'epilepsy day' bemoan the stigmatisation and they are right to do so. Nevertheless, the fact that the articles exist and the fact that there are 'epilepsy days' show how public perception has changed over the period. We must not be complacent, and much still needs to be done, and furthermore, societal attitudes can change quickly. However, what might be called the institutionalised stigma of the years between 1860 and 1960 is a thing of the past, at least in Europe and the United States, and legislation now protects those with epilepsy rather than renders them vulnerable; inclusion is preached, not exclusion. Stigma still exists but the various serious measures taken against the person of people with epilepsy have ceased. The situation in the developing world is probably far less good, although surveys are few, but stigma and disadvantage still play a major role in many impoverished people with epilepsy in low-income settings in Africa and Asia. The solution may be better education and there are many active public health campaigns to demystify the condition and reduce its secondary handicap.

However, in Western countries at least, the situation is far better than it was even 40 years ago. This is why we believe the modification of social attitudes around epilepsy in the last 40 years to be the greatest improvement for patients with epilepsy in the modern era.

Notes

1. Sir Edward Henry Sieveking (1816–1904) was a renowned early neurologist. His book (1) was a classic of early epileptology.
2. Bénédict Augustin Morel (1809–1873) was a leading French psychiatrist. His theories of degeneration were propounded in his book (2).
3. This gloomy prediction was part of much wider public concerns about social disintegration and the collapsing state of European culture, particularly in the face of the growth in cities, and the urban working class living in squalor and who had more offspring and reproduced younger than the respectable middle and upper classes. There were many in the privileged classes, all over Europe, who were concerned that the vigour of the European population was deteriorating, and that rapid population growth among the peasant and lower classes would sap national intelligence and morality.
4. Cesare Lombroso (1835–1909) was an Italian physician and criminologist. He wrote about epilepsy and criminality in various parts of his oeuvre, including in his famous book *L'uomo delinquente* (Milan, Hoepli) which went through five editions between 1876 and 1896/7.
5. Sir Francis Galton FRS (1822–1911).
6. Tallis explores the contemporary neuroscience scene in his devastating critique of what he amusingly calls neuromania and Darwinitis (8).
7. Action T4 was so-called because the office coordinating the killing was T4-Zentraldienststelle in Tiergartenstrasse 4, Berlin.
8. Among the three top experts for adult patients was Werner Heyde, Professor of Neurology and Psychiatry at the University of Würzburg, who kept his Chair while he was organising the killing of patients. He was identified in 1947 but was able to escape and was recaptured 12 years later, having been working as a physician under a different name, and charged with manslaughter in 1964. He committed suicide by hanging in his prison cell in 1964. Among the three experts for children was Werner Catel (1894–1961) who was Professor and Chair for Pediatrics at Leipzig University. Some researchers believe that Catel alone approved the killing of a total of 5000 children. Catel was never convicted of any crime and continued undisturbed as a Professor of Pediatrics until he retired on his own wish as Chair of Pediatrics at Christian-Albrechts-University Kiel (Germany) in 1960.

References

1. **Sieveking E.** *Epilepsy and Epileptiform Seizures: Their Causes, Pathology and Treatment.* London: John Churchill; 1858.
2. **Morel BA.** *Traité des dégénérescences physiques, intellectuelles et morales de l'espèce humaine et des causes qui produisent ces variétés maladives.* Paris: Baillière; 1857.

3. **Turner WA.** *Epilepsy: A Study of the Idiopathic Disease.* London: Macmillan & Company; 1907.
4. **Clark LP.** *Clinical Studies in Epilepsy.* New York: State Hospitals Press; 1917.
5. **Lennox W, Lennox M.** *Epilepsy and Related Disorders.* Boston, MA: Little Brown; 1960.
6. **Davenport CB, Weeks DF.** A first study of inheritance of epilepsy. *J Nerv Ment Dis* 1911; **38**:641–670.
7. **Lombardo PA.** Three generations, no imbeciles: new light on Buck v. Bell. *N Y Univ Law Rev* 1985; **60**(1):30–62.
8. **Tallis R.** *Aping Mankind: Neuromania, Darwinitis and the Misrepresentation of Humanity.* Durham: Acumen; 2011.
9. **Goffman I.** *Stigma.* London: Pelican Books; 1970.
10. **Alkhamees HA, Selai C, Shorvon S.** The beliefs amongst patients with epilepsy in Saudi Arabia about the causes and treatment of epilepsy, and other aspects. *Epilepsy Behav* 2015; **53**:135–139.
11. **de Boer HM.** *How to Measure and Reduce Stigma & the Experience from Other Conditions.* n.d. [Online] http://www.epilepsyallianceeurope.org/_fileupload/1%20-%20BurdenStigma%20of%20Epilepsy%20-%20Hanneke%20de%20Boer.pdf
12. **Jacoby A, Gorry J, Gamble C, Baker GA.** Public knowledge, private grief: a study of public attitudes to epilepsy in the United Kingdom and implications for stigma. *Epilepsia* 2004; **45**:1405–1415.
13. **Baker GA, Brooks J, Buck D, Jacoby A.** The stigma of epilepsy: a European perspective. *Epilepsia* 2000; **41**:98–104.
14. **Clinical Standards Advisory Group.** *Services for People with Epilepsy.* London: Department of Health; 2000.

Chapter 3

The Pharmaceutical Phoenix Rises

The history of drug treatment in the period 1860–1970 is one dominated by five drugs: at the beginning by bromide first mooted as an antiepileptic in 1857, and in widespread use by 1864, and at the end by valproate, licensed first in 1967. In between were the landmark discoveries of phenobarbital[1] in 1912, phenytoin in 1936, and carbamazepine licensed in 1962. These five compounds changed the lives of people with epilepsy, more perhaps than any other treatments and deserve to be celebrated. Each though was a child of its time, and here their story and its lessons, unflattering at times, will be briefly told. Landmarks yes, but a cure no.

The 1860s were a period of turmoil. Europe was embroiled in revolution, there were outbreaks of war in Europe, South America, and in Australasia, and in America a civil war. It was a decade, too, of scientific and technological advance, and of political and social reform. A scientific revolution was taking place in medicine, the germ theory of disease became established, Lister invented antisepsis, Galton developed theories of inheritance, Snow founded concepts of public health, and Florence Nightingale started the first school of nursing. In this period, too, the organisation of medical care was taking a shape that would be recognisable today, medical education was modernised, and medicine itself was becoming more internationalised. In Britain, for example, the Medical Act of 1858 created an official council for better regulation of doctors and to compile a pharmacopoeia in which there should be 'a list of medicines and compounds, and the manner of preparing them, and the true weights and measures by which they are prepared and mixed'. These were the stirrings of regulation in an area previously largely unregulated.

The First Effective Drugs

In the field of epilepsy therapy, too, the phoenix was beginning to rise. Until this time, the medicinal treatment of epilepsy, as with all other medical conditions, was mostly by 'empirics' as opposed to 'specifics'. Delasiauve divided therapy in his *Traité de l'épilepsie* of 1854, into (i) debilitating therapies (such as bleeding, tepid baths); (ii) evacuant therapies (including emetics and purgatives); (iii) sedative therapies (including ether); and (iv) specifics (including valerian and opiates) which he considered largely ineffective, and this was the common view.[2]

Sieveking published the first monograph on epilepsy in the modern era in 1857, with a second edition in 1861 in which he devoted 88 pages to treatment (4). He took what today would be called a holistic approach, with advice about hygiene, diet, rest, employment, education, intellectual pursuits, and moral instruction. Most of his medicinal therapeutics was aimed at treating the fit in the acute phase or preventing the development of the seizure in the premonitory phase and he recommended the use of counterirritation by terebinthinate, fomentations, or sinapisms; removal of all restraint; avoidance of sedatives, ammonia, and volatile stimulants; cool air; carotid compression; cold applications; galvanism; chloroform ligatures to the extremities; leeches to the temple; dry cupping; and the abstraction of blood (by various means). He reported that surgical amputation of the arm in which the aura develops, or removal of a testicle had been used successfully and, with more evident enthusiasm, trephination. In terms of chronic medicinal treatment, he recognised the inutility of most of these, but mentions counterirritants, purgatives, mineral tonics, nitro-muriatic acid, gentian, decoction of bark and sulphuric acid, and oleum morrhuae. He remained sceptical about the use of specifics, as he put it:

> I make these remarks not only as an apology for not entering more fully into the consideration of a host of drugs that may be used in the course of the treatment of epilepsy with more or less advantage; but also as a protest against that specialism, fostered by the public as well as the profession, which converts every disease into a separate entity, breaks up the unity of the science of medicine, and, in its extremes, does more harm than any extra-professional quackery.

He listed therapies he found generally unhelpful and these included opiates and narcotics, hyoscine, conium, belladonna, hydrocyanic acid, digitalis, mistletoe, cotyledon umbilicus, and indigo, and ended his chapter on treatment with his famous aphorism: 'In fact, there is not a substance in the material medica, there is scarcely a substance in the world, capable of passing through the gullet of man, that has not at one time or other enjoyed a reputation of being an anti-epileptic'.

At this time, most drugs were plant derivatives, animal derivatives, or simple chemicals. The plant and animal extracts were produced largely in local pharmacies and dispensaries, and were entirely unregulated (Table 3.1). The herbal remedies were extremely varied. Many have undoubted psychotropic and non-psychotropic actions and some at least of the large number of remedies have since been shown to have mild antiepileptic activity.[3] Animal-based extracts

Table 3.1 Herbal, animal, and chemical remedies for epilepsy in the nineteenth century

Herbal	Aconite (wolf's bane), *Adonis vernalis, Bryonia, Cannabis,* calabar bean, *Conium* (hemlock), *Cotyledon umbilicus* (penny wort), ergot, *Digitalis, Gelsemium sempervirens* (yellow jasmine), hydrastine, indigo, mistletoe, opium (and codeia), picrotoxin (from *Connulus indicus*), *Piscidia erthrina* (fishfuddle), rue, santonin (artemisia), *Selinum* (marsh parsley), simulo (hyssop), *Solanum carolinense* (nightshade), *Strophanthus,* strychnine, valerian. Also, extracts of the *Solonaceae* (nightshade) family: atropine, belladonna, hyacine, *Solanum carolinense,* stomonium
Animal	Crotalin (rattlesnake venom), curare, thyroidin, toxins, and anti-serum
Chemical	Amylene hydrate, borax, coal-tar (acetanilide, phenacetin, acetophenetidin), chinolin (quinoline), copper sulphate, chloral hydrate, chloralamide, chloretone, iron, nitroglycerine, osmic acid, pepto-mangan, potassium iodide, resorcin, sodium eosinate, silver nitrate, sulphonal, urethane, zinc (oxide, sulphate, acetate, valerianate, lactate, nitrate)

Adapted with permission from Shorvon SD, Historical introduction. In: *Treatment of Epilepsy,* 4th edition, Shorvon SD, Perucca E, Engel J (eds.), Oxford: Wiley-Blackwell. Copyright © 2015 John Wiley and Sons.

included toxins and venoms and could be used only very cautiously. As the modern era proceeded, however, it was the synthetic chemical remedies, led by bromide, which were to become predominant and in the end were to replace all others in the doctor's bag.

On the evening of 11 May 1857, a remarkable meeting was held at the London Royal Medical and Chirurgical Society (5). Here Sieveking gave a paper outlining his holistic approach, recommending the use of counterirritants, the promotion of healthy action of the secernent organs (secreting organs), and the value of vegetable and metallic roborants (tonics). Sieveking's talk was followed by a comment by Sir Charles Locock, Queen Victoria's obstetrician, that he had used potassium bromide with dramatic success in hysterical catamenial epilepsy (he also advised the removing of over-crowded teeth and the cessation of masturbation). In the 1961 edition of his book, Sieveking mentions that he had, following this meeting, tried bromide and 'though I have not enjoyed the same amount of success [as Sir Charles], I have found it decidedly beneficial. In one case, where the irritation of the sexual apparatus was very marked, a permanent cure seemed to be attributable to it'.

Thus, with a focus on onanism, was started a revolution in the therapy of epilepsy, with repercussions in many fields, and the beginning of a long series of synthetic medicinal discoveries which came to dominate treatment. These chemical remedies were produced at that stage largely by chemical and dye-making companies which were in the later years of the nineteenth century starting to be organised into a proto-pharmaceutical industry. In Germany, particularly, these companies began devoting increasing resources to research and development, but the science and manufacturing processes were still at a primitive stage. An entertaining description of a typical manufacturing outfit of the period, the May and Baker Garden Wharf factory in London, was published in 1889 (cited in 6):

> So we passed straight away into a land of huge retorts and seething furnaces, I was amused with the sight of an iron weight which I could not lift floating buoyantly in a lake of mercury. I choked in the camphor making sheds, which when they periodically catch fire, have simply to be left to burn down and a rare blaze they make. I shuddered as noxious compounds like corrosive sublimate and nitric acid and other *diableries*, to which vitriol is to mothers milk, were dealt with around me by the hogshead and the hundredweight. I was shown a huge tank of pure ether and on holding my hand under a tap was given the sensation of clinging to an iceberg at the North Pole.

Such factories produced the raw chemical of bromide which was then bought by the hospital pharmacies, which formulated them for dispensing. By 1899, bromides were widely used, and at the National Hospital for the Paralysed and the Epileptic at Queen Square in London, for instance, nearly two tons of bromide were being dispensed annually in the hospital pharmacy.

Within a short time, a variety of different bromide formulations appeared in clinical practice—these included bromide of aluminium, ammonium, potassium, sodium, lithium, strontium, nickel, camphor, rubidium and ammonium, iodine, chorine, bromaline (bromine and formaldehyde derivatives), bromapin (bromine and seseme oil), hydrobromic acid, and Gélineau's formula (bromide and arsenic). All tasted vile, and so other ingredients were added, such as syrup of Virginian prune which was a favourite of Gowers. By 1914, there were 45 different formulations, each of which had their advocates, but most of which were considered by Aldren Turner[4], one of the leading epileptologist of the time, as 'quack formulations'. The reasons for this proliferation were no doubt commercial, and perhaps too they allowed some doctors to claim unique therapies not available to others; in the history of epilepsy, it is an early example of me-too multiplication which was to remain an all-too-prevalent tendency in later years.

Bromides were undoubtedly effective, and positive trials of bromide continue to be reported right up the present day. It is their side effects though which limit their use. These were recognised early and the constellation of effects became known as 'bromism' and was an ominous state of affairs. Turner in 1907 (7) provides a vivid description:

> This condition [bromism] is characterised by a blunting of the intellectual faculties, impairment of the memory, and the production of a dull and apathetic state. The speech is slow, the tongue tremulous and saliva may flow from the mouth. The gait

is staggering, and the movements of the limbs feeble and infirm. The mucous membranes suffer, so that the palatal sensibility may be abolished, and nausea, flatulence, and diarrhoea supervene. The action of the heart is low and feeble, the respiration shallow and imperfect, and the extremities blue and cold. An eruption of acne frequently covers the skin of the face and back.

The skin lesions, in their fullest form, were known as 'bromoderma' with boils, pustules, and weeping sores sometimes requiring surgical treatment. Psychiatric symptoms such as disinhibition, self-neglect, irritability, violent behaviour, emotional instability, depression, and occasionally a schizophrenic-like psychosis were reported and hallucinations were not uncommon. Turner believed correctly that the side effects occurred mainly when the dose was too high, and that skilful treatment could minimise these; nevertheless, bromide-soaked individuals in back-wards of asylums became synonymous with 'epileptics' and the drug side effects added to the stigma of the condition discussed in Chapter 2.

Turner's book is now recognised as a classic in the epilepsy literature, and it is interesting to see his observations on other therapies. He was at pains to emphasise that 'no greater mistake can be made in the treatment of epilepsy than to rely solely on medicinal means, which so often fail to gain the desired end … We have, therefore, in every case of epilepsy to treat the individual and not solely the disease' and he was a keen advocate of institutional care, and measures to improve employment, education, and emotional life. In relation to drugs, he was dismissive of most of the herbal remedies previously recommended, and the only drugs other than bromides he thought especially effective were chloral hydrate, borax, and belladonna (with zinc, opium, strychnine, atropine, and tonics sometimes useful). He devoted a page of his book to 'miscellaneous methods of treatment' which included 'organotherapy', the administration of thyroid or thymus gland or cerebrin, the latter being obtained from brain and nerve tissue, and 'serotherapy', the injection of blood serum from either another epileptic or the same epileptic; but was not impressed by either. Constipation was a preoccupation of all epilepsy doctors of the period, and Turner, as all others, recommended enemas, laxatives, and even occasional colectomy. As he wrote: 'Epileptics are notoriously big eaters, and being habitually subject to constipation, are prone to overload the digestive tracts and organs'. He was interested in diets, especially the purine-free diet, and physical and mental hygiene. The physician should specify 'the proper allotment of work and rest, and the carrying out of those physical and mental exercises consistent with the malady'. He noted the beneficial effects of daily exercise in the open air, hot baths, spinal douches, and massage, the avoidance of alcohol and the disparagement of marriage. As for employment, 'an outdoor life is usually regarded as most suitable … but there are many semi-sedentary forms of work suitable for the frailer epileptic such as drawing, modelling, and office work, bookkeeping and the like'. He wrote also on the management of education of children which he felt should be tailored to individual capabilities, as he wrote 'no greater mistake is committed in the management of young epileptics, than withholding from them the advantages of the mental and physical exercises entailed by educational methods under special supervision and direction'. This was the state of epilepsy therapeutics in the early twentieth century, but in 1912, all began to change.

The discovery of the antiepileptic effect of phenobarbital, in 1912, was the landmark in therapy and one of those classic stories in the epilepsy canon. At that time, phenobarbital was one of a family of barbiturates licensed and marketed as a sleeping draught (a hypnotic is the technical term) by the German chemical company Bayer, under the trade name Luminal. Dr Alfred Hauptmann, then a junior psychiatrist in Freiburg, thought of giving phenobarbital to his epilepsy patients to help them sleep, as the noise of their fits kept him awake at night. He then noted to his surprise that both the frequency and the severity of the epileptic seizures were greatly reduced. He published his findings in an article in 1912 (8) in which he had carefully recorded the effect on seizures over a period of months so as to avoid being misled by random fluctuations, and at different doses (maximum 300 mg/day). He concluded that phenobarbital was effective in even the severest cases of epilepsy for which bromide was ineffective. He presented a case history of a patient in whom Luminal had been substituted for bromide, who not only had fewer seizures but whose mental agility and 'state of nutrition and strength improved to a quite extraordinary degree'. In 1919, he extended his observations (9) and then recommended phenobarbital for treatment of 'genuine' epilepsy and also status epilepticus. These papers were landmarks in the field, but initially largely overlooked by the wider epilepsy community, perhaps because they appeared in a German-language journal at a time when war was being joined, but in the 1920s, following further reports from England and the United States, phenobarbital use rapidly spread around the world. Its great effectiveness meant that by the 1930s and 1940s it was generally considered the drug of first choice in epilepsy (Box 3.1). Hauptmann's life was itself eventful. He was awarded an Iron Cross for services in the First World War, became Professor of Psychiatry in Halle, Germany, but was then incarcerated in Dachau concentration camp in the Second World War, then emigrated to the United Kingdom and finally to the United States where he died in 1948.

One striking feature of antiepileptic drug therapy is how long it takes for side effects to be recognised. This was indeed the case with phenobarbital.

> **Box 3.1 Drugs in common use for epilepsy in 1940**
>
> - Bromide (in any of the following salts: sodium, potassium, ammonium, lithium, calcium, calcium bromine galactogluconate)
> - Bromide combinations
> - Phenobarbitone (luminal)
> - *N*-methylethylphenylmalonyl urea (Prominal)
> - Borax
> - Belladonna (sometimes with bromide or bromide and caffeine)
> - Nitroglycerine (sometimes with strychnine and bromide)
> - Dialacetin (a mixture of the hypnotic allobarbital (Dial) with allylparacetaminophenol).
>
> Source: data from Wilson SAK. *Neurology*, London: Edward Arnold, Copyright © 1940 Taylor and Francis.

Although it had been quickly noted that high doses could cause sedation, it was claimed that at lower doses in epilepsy, the drug 'cleared the mentality'. In fact, this effect was not due to the phenobarbital, but to the concomitant reduction in bromide dosage but it turned out to be a useful marketing slogan. Not least as sedation was then almost sine qua non of life for an epilepsy sufferer. Some other neurotoxic effects such as incoordination, visual disturbance, and ataxia were identified by 1920, as was the risk of severe exacerbation of seizures if the drug was withdrawn too rapidly. However, other side effects evaded early detection. The potential for dependency was noted only in the 1940s, and hypersensitivity, effects on folate, vitamin K, osteomalacia, and the shoulder hand syndrome, knee- and hip pain, thickening of the footsoles and the penis and paradoxical excitement in children were all identified only after 40–50 years of clinical use. It was only in 1979 that the way phenobarbital exerts its antiepileptic action, by binding to brain gamma-aminobutyric acid (GABA) receptors, was discovered.

Phenobarbital has an interesting societal as well as medical history. In the 1950s and 1960s, phenobarbital had become widely prescribed for any condition in which 'stress' was thought contributory, such as migraine, hypertension, asthma, and panic attacks. This led to considerable over-prescription. Then, in the 1950s and 1960s, many psychotropic agents started to be misused and in the midst of this haze of abuse was phenobarbital (Box 3.2). It became a street drug and the cause of many cases of addiction, dependency, and fatal overdose.

Barbiturate 'goofballs' were handed out to US troops in the Pacific in the 1950s and it is still claimed that 9% of all Americans have misused barbiturate at some point in their lives. This has led to efforts to regulate its manufacture, distribution, and prescription and in 1971 the United Nations designated phenobarbital as a controlled substance. Despite these problems, it remains a remarkably cheap drug to manufacture, and so today continues to be widely used to treat epilepsy in the developing world and is included in the WHO *Essential Drugs List* for this purpose. Its low cost though means that the major pharmaceutical companies have no interest in producing it, and this and the bureaucracies of its status as a controlled substance have resulted in problems of supply and distribution in many developing countries. No manufacturer provides any marketing or promotion, in contrast to the huge marketing budgets of other pharmaceutical products. Its extreme cheapness and simplicity of manufacture would in a rational world be considered an advantage, but no such advantage can be realised in the marketing-driven environment of modern therapeutics. However, it does remain in the formularies, and indeed phenobarbital is one of only 12 pre-First World War medicaments in the current *British National Formulary*, and most of the others are now rarely prescribed. When the WHO recommendation to use phenobarbital was first made, Fritz Dreifuss, the then ILAE President, disagreed with the policy, saying that to use phenobarbital in resource-poor settings, but not in Western countries, puts 'a hierarchy on the brain' and that people in resource-poor countries were being consigned to second-class medication. WHO, however, carried out a meta-analysis in 2002 showing that there was no evidence that phenobarbital was any less effective than newer antiepileptics. This is a difficult and thorny issue, and the equation is not as simple as Dreifuss suggested, where cost, availability, safety, and efficacy all enter the mix.

In the 1920s and 1930s, although phenobarbital and bromide dominated therapy, other drugs such as borax, belladonna, and zinc were also sometimes recommended. Interestingly, in 2006, a new study of borax was published showing quite reasonable effectiveness but this is one drug which seems now to have totally fallen from use anywhere in the world. A curious zinc formulation was zinc bread which was made in the late nineteenth century but failed to catch on as its taste was apparently disgusting. Nevertheless, zinc remains a popular alternative-medicine choice for epilepsy today. Various new barbiturates were also formulated, on the me-too principle of drug production. A range of other therapies also came and went in the 1930s, amongst the strangest (and colourful) of which were the 'vital dyes' brilliant red and methyl blue, and rattle-snake venom.

La Nouvelle Vague

Of course, the landmark discovery, which overshadowed all others in this period, was that of phenytoin. It is a story that has been repeatedly told and is not gone into again here in any detail, but it does have some lessons for us today. In Boston, Massachusetts, the neurologists Merrit and Putnam, were given the drug by Parke-Davis, the pharmaceutical company, and tested it in their new 'maximal electrical shock model' which involved administering increasingly strong electric currents to cats, restrained in a box, via scalp and mouth electrodes. When the electrical current was strong enough, a convulsion was precipitated, and this was defined as the 'threshold' current. The drug was then administered and the experiment repeated to see if a higher threshold current was needed to produce a seizure. In this way, the antiepileptic effect of a drug could be quantified (i.e. by the increase in current needed) and drugs compared. Phenytoin was one of the first drugs tried, first in 1936, and the results were published in the 28 May issue of *Science* in 1937 (10). Preliminary findings of eight patients were then reported in August 1937, and the results of the first clinical trial unveiled in June 1938 at the annual meeting of the American Medical Association. By 1939 there were 13 open case series reported and by 1940 the drug was in wide usage around the world (11–14). This extraordinarily rapid take-up of the drug was partly due to the muscular advertising of Parke-Davis who had adverts and publicity inserted into medical journals and the public media. Indeed, this was the first example in epilepsy of the use of extensive marketing by the pharmaceutical industry, and it proved very successful.

In 1945, Merritt and Putnam had published the results of testing of over 700 compounds using their experimental method, of which four were selected for clinical trial (15). This was the first time that a really systematic approach was taken to screen compounds, and now mass animal screening is part of the developmental programme of all the major pharmaceutical companies. It is a matter of irony that it is now accepted that Merritt and Putnam's method does not reliably measure seizure threshold, and furthermore, phenytoin does not actually reliably increase threshold, but such is the history of epilepsy drug development. One spin-off of the screening though was the discovery of the drug ethosuximide which although having a structure close to that of phenytoin, does not in fact have an effect in partial epilepsy, but was found by chance to be useful in absence seizures (another form of epilepsy) and it continues to be used today, with no drug shown to have superior efficacy. It was one of a series of succinimide drugs licensed then, but the others proved too toxic for use and so have subsequently been phased out.

Phenytoin was not a sedative to the same extent as phenobarbital and bromide, and this was partly the reason for its rapid success, and following its introduction, the use of bromide (and belladonna and borax) tailed off dramatically, and phenytoin and phenobarbital became the two undisputed aces in the antiepileptic pack. The many side effects of phenytoin were slowly and progressively recognised over the next 20 years, and indeed the drug became the example to test when any new pharmaceutical side effect was postulated, and it usually did not disappoint. The first inkling of damaging effects on the fetus, when mothers take phenytoin during pregnancy, was first reported in 1968 but the extent of this problem was recognised only some decades later. Also, its remarkable non-linear metabolism, which results in unexpectedly high increases in the amount of the drug circulating in the body after only very small dose increases, became a paradigmatic model for pharmacokinetic studies. Indeed, the introduction of 'therapeutic drug monitoring' was largely due to the need for serum phenytoin level estimations to guide clinical practice, and phenytoin still remains the drug for which such monitoring is most helpful. Despite all its manifest problems, phenytoin remains a drug widely used for epilepsy even today, partly because of its cheapness (only phenobarbital costs less) and partly because prescribing practice in epilepsy is very conservative. The notion of 'better the devil you know' is very strongly held, with some justification as experience with later drugs was to show, but phenytoin certainly is no angel.

Its mechanism of action, the blockage of the neuronal sodium channel, was discovered in 1983 and this too was a landmark discovery in field of drug physiology and marked the beginning of a wave of intense interest in channel function in epilepsy which has yielded many dividends. This and the discovery of phenobarbital's action on the GABA receptors in the brain were the first time that the contemporary advances in molecular biology applied to study of antiepileptic drug mechanisms of action, and thenceforward drugs began to be purposely designed to affect specific molecular targets. In the past, the introduction of treatment was sometimes grounded in contemporary theories of causation—for instance, bromide on the basis that this might reduce masturbation by its effects on sexual excitation, the use of colectomy to counter 'autointoxication', counterirritation methods to damp down reflexes, or carotid ligation to reduce excessive blood flow. Many others were introduced on a me-too basis including the 45 types of bromide and the even greater number of barbiturate, benzodiazepine, and hydantoin variants. Indeed, Parke-Davis had originally synthesised phenytoin in their search for hypnotic drugs on the basis that the hydantoins had ring structures similar to that of the barbiturates. Most drugs, however, were the product of chance findings, although sometimes justified post hoc by retrospective theorising, and it was this so-called serendipity which marked the discovery of the next two landmark drugs in epilepsy, carbamazepine and valproate (Box 3.2).

The next decade, between 1958 and 1968, was certainly the most important in the history of drug treatment for epilepsy.[5] A range of new drugs was

Box 3.2 The drugs used in the treatment of epilepsy in 1955, derived from the international list of antiepileptic drugs published in *Epilepsia*

Barbiturates

- Phenylethyl barbituric acid
- Phenylethyl malonylurea
- Methylphenyl barbituric acid
- Methylphenylethyl barbituric acid
- Methyldiethyl barbituric acid.

Combinations with barbiturate:

- Phenylethyl barbituric acid, belladonna, and caffeine
- Phenylethyl barbituric acid and amphetamine.

Oxazolidine diones

- Trimethyl oxazolidine dione
- Dimethylethyl oxazolidine dione
- Diphenyl oxazolidine dione
- Allylmethyl oxazolidine dione.

Hydantoins

- Diphenyl hydantoin (or diphenyl hydantoin sodium)
- Methyldiphenyl hydantoin
- Methylphenylethyl hydantoin
- Methyldibromophenylethyl hydantoin
- Dimethyldithio hydantoin
- Sodium phenylthienyl hydantoin
- Methylphenyl hydantoin.

Combinations with hydantoins:
- Diphenyl hydantoin and phenobarbital
- Diphenyl hydantoin, phenobarbital, and caffeine
- Diphenyl hydantoin, phenobarbital, and desoxyephedrine
- Methylphenylethylhydantoin and phenobarbital
- Diphenyl hydantoin and methylphenylethyl barbituric acid
- Diphenyl hydantoin, methylphenylethyl barbituric acid, and phenobarbital.

Other types
- Phenylacetylurea
- Phenylethylhexahydropyrimidine dione
- Benzchlorpropamide
- Methylalphaphenyl succinimide
- Acetazolamide
- Alkaline borotartrates
- Glutamic acid (or glutamic acid-HCl)
- Bromides.

Source: data from International list of anti-epilepsy drugs, *Epilepsia*, Volume C4, Issue 1, pp. 121–3, Copyright © 1955 ILAE.

introduced which included ethosuximide and the benzodiazepines; however, it was carbamazepine and valproate which were to prove to have the greatest importance in the long-term treatment of epilepsy. Carbamazepine, initially known as G32883, was developed in the Swiss pharmaceutical company Geigy in 1953. As it had a structure similar to tricyclic antidepressants, it was investigated first for action in depression and psychosis for which it appeared to have disappointingly little effect, and then for neuropathic pain where its effects were noted to be quite strong. It was in fact licensed for trigeminal neuralgia in 1962 and is still widely used in this excruciating and debilitating form of nerve pain. Its antiepileptic effects, found largely by chance, were first reported in 1963, and carbamazepine was licensed for epilepsy first in 1965 (Figure 3.1). The early trials[6] continued to explore its potential to improve mood as well as control seizures, and this potential property was made much of in the corporate promotions of the drug at the time, although as the smoke has cleared, it

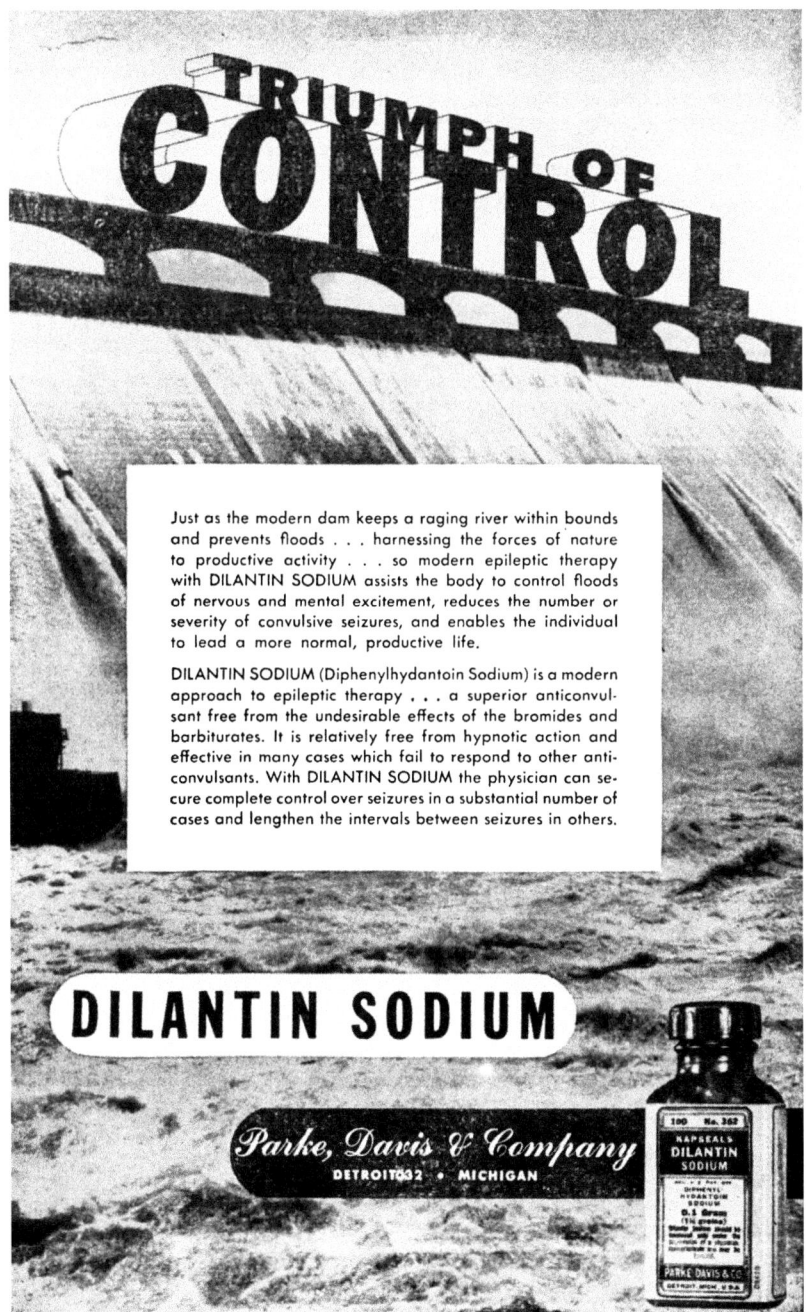

Figure 3.1 An early advertisement for phenytoin, by its original manufacturer. Reproduced by kind permission of Pfizer. Copyright © 2016 Pfizer Inc. All rights reserved.

seems apparent that the mood-enhancing properties of carbamazepine are relatively weak. It is not a sedative, and this was a distinct advantage, and within only 10 years of its introduction, it had become very widely used, especially in Europe. Indeed, 50 years later, it is still a drug of first choice in the treatment of most of the common forms of epilepsy. No subsequent antiepileptic drug has been shown conclusively to be superior and carbamazepine has in many ways become the gold standard treatment, especially in partial epilepsy, against which all opposition is pitched. It was promoted as less sedative than phenytoin, ironically so as phenytoin was itself initially promoted as a drug without sedation, and skilfully marketed. The drug changed hands as the drug companies became involved in complex mergers with Tegretol owed initially by Geigy, then Ciba-Geigy, then Novartis[7], and these companies became prominent sponsors of medical conferences and meetings and had a large sales forces promoting the drug in doctors' surgeries all over the world. Thus, carbamazepine became the first antiepileptic drug to fully enter the booming pharmaceutical market of the 1970s, and was the first to make large profits for its manufacturer. The main drawback of carbamazepine, from the clinical point of view, is its side effects. A serious rash may occasionally occur and very rarely allergic reactions resulting in liver or bone marrow failure, and these and the other commoner but less serious side effects of the drug were identified by the end of the 1960s. Fifty years later, carbamazepine remains the most investigated antiepileptic on the market, and it is now so well studied that many consider it to be the safest of the current antiepileptics and the one with least potential to surprise; in the conservative world of neurological therapeutics, this is a reassuring profile.

The next drug to mention is valproate. The antiepileptic value of this drug was a totally unexpected finding, and this is another well-known story in the canon of epilepsy therapeutics. Valproic acid had been used for over 80 years as an organic solvent, and was being used for this purpose in a small pharmaceutical laboratory in Grenoble by three young scientists, P. Eymard and the brothers H. and Y. Meunier in the testing of a series of compounds for tranquillising action in the rat in 1962. When all the compounds were found to be active, the brothers decided to test the solvent alone and found it to be a remarkably effective antiepileptic. They then studied the drug in 16 rabbits given the convulsant cardiazol, and in the same year it was given in a trial run to 16 patients.[8] Thirteen of the 16 cases showed marked improvement in the study, and as it became rapidly apparent that this small laboratory could not provide the resources for a major development programme, the drug was sold to Sanofi, the French pharmaceutical company. In 1967, it received its first human licence, and like carbamazepine soon became widely used, especially in Europe. In the United States, the regulatory agencies were less compliant, possibly because, it has been claimed, it was not an American drug, and licensing was initially withheld. Kiffin Penry, the ILAE President at the time, then led a campaign to the US Senate seeking access for US citizens for the drug and eventually the drug was licensed in 1976, albeit only for the treatment of absence seizures. The whole battle for approval of valproate was dramatised in a 1987 ABC television film, *Fight for Life*, and seen as an example of the arbitrariness of regulatory approval and the essentially political nature of many of these decisions.[9]

Valproate is a drug which has especial value in types of seizures (absence and myoclonic seizures) not treated by carbamazepine or phenytoin, and a type of epilepsy known as 'Idiopathic Generalised Epilepsy'. This is a common form of epilepsy and the lack of sedation made valproate an immediately popular drug, and its introduction led to a rapid fall in the previously widespread prescription of phenytoin. The main drawbacks of valproate are its side effects, notably weight gain and tremor. It occasionally causes a severe 'encephalopathy' (with stupor or even coma), may elevate ammonia levels in the blood to dangerous levels, and has resulted in pancreatic or liver failure. It has also been shown to cause hormonal disorders in women, and possibly polycystic ovarian syndrome. These effects are bad enough but the looming concern in recent years has been over its effects on the unborn child if given to women during pregnancy. The first such problems were noted in 1982 when a higher than normal rate of spinal bifida was noted and then in the 1980s and 1990s children exposed to valproate were found sometimes to have a 'fetal syndrome' consisting of bone and skeletal abnormalities and also learning disability. It was in 2001, though, that the first studies were published which looked specifically at whether valproate exposure in pregnancy might result in subsequent learning disability in the offspring. In fact, there appears to be a significant risk and it has been only in the last few years that this has been adequately quantified. What is a salutary lesson is that it has taken 50 years for these effects to be clearly identified and one wonders how many children were born in earlier years with disadvantages because of this drug. In 2015, the European regulatory authority suggested that valproate should not be used in women of childbearing age, but the epilepsy community has reacted against this suggestion, largely because of the undisputed clear superiority of valproate for controlling seizures in Idiopathic Generalised Epilepsy. Thus, doctors and patients are in a difficult position, where risks and benefits have to be carefully weighed. Of course this is true for all treatments in all situations, but for valproate in young adult women with Idiopathic Generalised Epilepsy, these therapy decisions have become particularly difficult.

In addition to valproate and carbamazepine, in the 1960s the development of benzodiazepines had a large impact on the treatment of acute seizures.[10]

They were interesting drugs, which had a much greater role in psychiatry. They indeed had a powerful impact on society and culture in the 1970s–1990s when diazepam ('mother's little helper'), for instance, had entered the folklore of the age. The discovery of these drugs fuelled a revolution in biological psychiatry and its social reaction. They were used in chronic epilepsy, but because of the tendency for the antiepileptic effects to wear off, and also the tendency for dependency of misuse, they are, with the exception of one compound, clobazam, not now used much in this role (Table 3.2).

The Rise of Big Pharma and, in Reaction, Regulation

A striking phenomenon in the history of epilepsy treatment in this period is the rise of the pharmaceutical industry. The industry first appeared in the late nineteenth century, emerging largely from chemical and dye-making companies, and initially there was modest growth. However, by the 1960s, the leading companies were making large profits and by a series of mergers and acquisitions became very large multinational corporations. A range of blockbuster drugs in other medical areas fuelled this growth in the 1950s and 1960s, and carbamazepine reaped the first such financial harvest in the area of epilepsy. This growth has had a number of consequences. The research ethos changed, and what was relatively open and transparent previously has become at least in the eyes of some critics much more commercially sensitive and competitive. The later stages of clinical development particularly have sometimes become a strictly commercial enterprise, with developments kept tightly under wraps to protect commercial interests. The marketing departments of the companies have also grown and increasingly sophisticated and powerful methods have been used to target doctors and consumers. The large profits and financial power of the companies have had some regrettable consequences. A series of lawsuits and scandals, concerned largely with marketing infringements, have plagued the industry and the public have become suspicious and nervous of the motives of the industry. None of this would have been predicted in the earlier period, when companies were rightly lauded for producing products of value to humanity.

In parallel with the increasing power of the industry, and in part a reaction against this, has been growing regulation and legislation designed to reign in the alleged excesses of the industry and to protect the public. As mentioned earlier, the first regulation of medicines in Britain was at the beginning of our story, in 1858, where the medical act required accurate labelling of content and quantity. In the United States in 1906, similar measures were taken. It was only in the 1930s that evidence of safety was required before drug licensing, in the United States, in

Table 3.2 Drugs used in the treatment of epilepsy between 1996 and 2014 (a listing of the chapters in the four editions of the textbook *The Treatment of Epilepsy*)

First edition, 1996	Second edition, 2004	Third edition, 2009	Fourth edition, 2016
	Acetazolamide	Acetazolamide	Acetazolamide
		Adrenocorticotropic hormone (ACTH) and corticosteroids	ACTH and corticosteroids
		Benzodiazepines used primarily for chronic treatment (clobazam, clonazepam, clorazepate, nitrazepam)	Benzodiazepines used in epilepsy (clobazam, clonazepam, clorazepate, diazepam, lorazepam, midazolam, nitrazepam)
Other benzodiazepines (clorazepate, diazepam, lorazepam, midazolam, nitrazepam)	Short-acting and other benzodiazepines (diazepam, lorazepam, midazolam, clorazepate, nitrazepam)	Benzodiazepines used primarily for emergency treatment (diazepam, lorazepam, midazolam)	
Carbamazepine and oxcarbazepine	Carbamazepine	Carbamazepine	Carbamazepine
Clobazam	Clobazam		
Clonazepam	Clonazepam		
	Fosphenytoin		
			Eslicarbazepine acetate
Ethosuximide and methsuximide	Ethosuximide	Ethosuximide	Ethosuximide
Felbamate	Felbamate	Felbamate	Felbamate
Gabapentin	Gabapentin	Gabapentin	Gabapentin
		Lacosamide	Lacosamide
Lamotrigine	Lamotrigine	Lamotrigine	Lamotrigine
	Levetiracetam	Levetiracetam	Levetiracetam

Table 3.2 Continued

First edition, 1996	Second edition, 2004	Third edition, 2009	Fourth edition, 2016
	Oxcarbazepine	Oxcarbazepine	Oxcarbazepine
			Perampanel
Phenobarbitone and primidone	Phenobarbital, primidone, and other barbiturates (metharbital, methylphenobarbital, barbexaclone)	Phenobarbital, primidone and other barbiturates	Phenobarbital, primidone and other barbiturates
Phenytoin	Phenytoin	Phenytoin	Phenytoin
Piracetam	Piracetam	Piracetam	Piracetam
	Pregabalin	Pregabalin	Pregabalin
			Retigabine
	Rufinamide	Rufinamide	Rufinamide
		Stiripentol	Stiripentol
	Tiagabine	Tiagabine	Tiagabine
Topiramate	Topiramate	Topiramate	Topiramate
Valproate	Valproate	Valproate	Valproate
Vigabatrin	Vigabatrin	Vigabatrin	Vigabatrin
	Zonisamide	Zonisamide	Zonisamide
Other drugs used in the treatment of epilepsy (acetazolamide, ACTH, allopurinol ethotoin, bromides, mephenytoin, paraldehyde, phenacemide, trimethadione)	Other drugs more rarely used in the treatment of epilepsy (ACTH, allopurinol. bromide, ethotoin, mephenytoin, paraldehyde, phenacemide, trimethadione)	Other drugs rarely used (allopurinol, bromide, ethotoin, furosemide, mephenytoin, phenacemide, trimethadione)	Other drugs rarely used (bromide, lidocaine, methsuximide, paraldehyde, sulthiame)

Source: data from Shorvon SD, Dreifuss F, Fish D, and Thomas D (eds). *The Treatment of Epilepsy*, 1st edition. Oxford: Blackwell Science Ltd., Copyright © 1996 Blackwell Science Ltd.; Shorvon SD, Dodson E, Fish DR, and Perucca E (eds). *The Treatment of Epilepsy*, 2nd edition. Oxford: Blackwell Science Ltd.; Shorvon SD, Perucca E, and Engel J (eds). *The Treatment of Epilepsy*, 3rd edition. Oxford: Wiley-Blackwell, Copyright © 2009 Wiley-Blackwell Ltd.; Shorvon SD, Perucca E, Engel J (eds). *The Treatment of Epilepsy*, 4th edition. Oxford: Wiley-Blackwell, Copyright © 2016 Wiley-Blackwell Ltd.

response to the scandal and public outrage caused by the deaths of more than 100 people caused by 'elixir of sulphanilamide', a liquid form of sulphanilamide, dissolved in diethylene glycol. The thalidomide tragedy of the 1950s then resulted in further tightening of the regulations by the US Food and Drug Administration (FDA) and the 1962 drugs act required evidence of efficacy as well as safety, the establishment of guidelines for testing, and a new system of licensing. This system remains in place. Complete chemical and manufacturing information, preclinical screening, and animal investigation, including toxicology, teratogenicity, and safety, are required to be submitted to the FDA before an investigatory licence is granted. Clinical testing is then divided into phase I (healthy volunteers), phase II (controlled studies in seizure patients), and phase III (broad and varied clinical studies) and after completion of these studies, a marketing and manufacturing licence can be applied for. This was a step-change in regulation. There have been some negative consequences. The cost of drug development has soared, the time taken to license a drug has been inordinately extended, and the number of drugs being tested has fallen. In the field of epilepsy, only the major companies now can afford to proceed, and although the public has been much more protected by the regulations, the downsides are appreciable. Whether we have the balance right now is highly arguable.

In addition to the drugs mentioned in this chapter, a whole host of other compounds were developed in this period, hailed with exaggerated claims but which have fallen from use because of what is eventually realised to be ineffectiveness or previously unrecognised side effects. This probably could have been avoided by better assessment methods than were used at the time, but the sharpest critics suspect, too, some claims made for new drugs in this period were exaggerated. This seems, in most cases, unlikely and the failure to characterise a drug reflects more the shaky nature of scientific mores and the fashions of the day (see Chapter 6). Regulations are much stricter, and the requirement to provide accurate information more strictly enforced, but nevertheless, this experience should encourage in all of us a degree of mild scepticism when we are now presented with similar assertions about contemporary therapies, which are themselves of course based on equally transient states of knowledge.

By 1970, drug discovery was moving from the age of structural chemistry into the age of molecular biology and a series of brilliant advances,[11] often due to new investigatory technologies, were having a great impact. It was then hoped that a new era of scientific target-based 'rational' therapy would follow, and advertisements celebrating the rationality of new drugs littered the journals (we are experiencing a rather similar pattern in relation to 'tailored' therapy, raised by, as some sceptical critics claim, the equally over-hyped claims of pharmacogenomics in epilepsy today). For the first time, drugs were being designed on the basis of molecular mechanisms, and there were surges of interest, for instance, in GABAergic mechanisms and in sodium and calcium channel blockade. At that time, seizures were felt to reflect an inadequate balance between excitation and inhibition in the brain, and were due either to excessive excitation or inadequate inhibition. Nevertheless, despite the new emphasis on science, almost all of the drugs discovered in this period were still the result of manipulation of the structure of existing compounds ('me-too' products) or of random screening or of pure chance. The failure of such 'designer' drugs to have an impact continues to this day and is one of the most disappointing aspects of epilepsy therapy.

The increase in regulation in the early 1960s and 1970s began to take its toll and over the next 15 years, very few new drugs were introduced. Things though were to change after 1989, when a new shoal of blockbuster drugs was introduced and when the sea again became alive with modern products. This period is the topic of Chapter 4, where many of the same issues relating to drug treatment, which have their origins in the nineteenth century, are again played out.

Notes

1. The drug was named phenobarbitone (the British Approved Name, BAN) and also phenobarbital (International Non-Proprietary Name, INN). The 2001–2003 EU harmonisation rules rationalised the usage and chose phenobarbital as the official name.
2. Many of the details of the history of drug treatment in the early period are taken from the following sources: Friedlander (1), Shorvon (2), and Lennox and Lennox (3).
3. For instance, valerian, aconite (wolf's bane), *Gelsemium sempervirens* (yellow jasmine), *Selinum* (marsh parsley), *Cannabis indica*, and the extracts of Solanaceae (the nightshade family) such as belladonna or atropine.
4. Turner was the leading epileptologist of his period. His book *Epilepsy: A Study of the Idiopathic Disease* (7) is recognised as a classic in the field and was republished in facsimile form by Raven Press, with an adulatory preface by J. Kiffin Penry in 1973.
5. For further details of the developments in this period, see Shorvon (16).
6. The first controlled trial was carried out after the drug was licensed, see Bird et al. (17).
7. The history of mergers in the pharmaceutical company is a fascinating example of the capitalism at the heart of the industry. The fate of the manufacturers of Tegretol is a good example. Geigy was founded as a chemicals and dyes company in 1901 and changed its name to J. R. Geigy in 1906. It merged with Ciba in 1971 to form Ciba-Geigy Ltd, and the company branched out into various chemical and pharmaceutical areas. In 1992, Ciba-Geigy was fined $62 million in the United States for illegal waste dumping, and in 1996, merged with Sandoz, to form Novartis. Sandoz was another chemical company, founded in Basel in 1886, which gained some notoriety as the marketer of LSD (under the name *Delysid*). In 1967, Sandoz merged with Wander AG, and in 1986, a fire in the Sandoz factory caused an environmental disaster as vast quantities of pesticide were released into

the Rhine. After this, it spun off its chemical branch and the pharmaceutical and agrochemical divisions merged with Ciba-Geigy to form Novartis.
8. For the discovery of valproate therapy, see Meunier et al. (18) and Carraz et al. (19).
9. For further details, see Shorvon (16).
10. For a history of the benzodiazepine drugs, see Sternbach (20).
11. For a study of the rise of modern neuroscience, see Shepherd (21).

References

1. **Friedlander WJ.** *The History of Modern Epilepsy: The Beginning, 1865–1914.* Westport, CT: Greenwood Press; 2001.
2. **Shorvon SD.** Drug treatment of epilepsy in the century of the ILAE: the first 50 years, 1909–1958. *Epilepsia* 2009; **50**(Suppl 3):69–92.
3. **Lennox WG, Lennox M.** *Epilepsy and Related Disorders.* Boston, MA: Little Brown; 1960.
4. **Sieveking EH.** *Epilepsy and Epileptiform Seizures: Their Causes, Pathology and Treatment*, 2nd ed. London: John Churchill; 1861.
5. **Anonymous.** Royal Medical and Chirurgical Society, Tuesday May 11th 1857. *Lancet* 1857; **1**:527–528.
6. **Slinn J.** Research and development in the UK pharmaceutical industry from the nineteenth century until the 1960s. In: Porter R Teich M (eds) *Drugs and Narcotics in History.* Cambridge: Cambridge University Press, 1995:168–186.
7. **Turner WA.** *Epilepsy: A Study of the Idiopathic Disease.* London: Macmillan and Co.; 1907.
8. **Hauptmann A.** Luminal bei Epilepsie. *Munch med Wochenschr* 1912; **59**:1907–1912.
9. **Hauptmann A.** Erfahrungen aus der Behandlung der Epilepsie mit Luminal. *Munch med Wochenschr* 1919; **46**:1319–1321.
10. **Putnam TJ, Merritt HH.** Experimental determination of the anticonvulsant properties of some phenyl derivatives. *Science* 1937; **85**:525–526.
11. **Merritt HH, Putnam TJ.** Sodium diphenyl hydantoinate in the treatment of convulsive disorders. *J Am Med Soc* 1938; **111**:1068–1073.
12. **Merritt HH, Putnam TJ.** Sodium diphenyl hydantoinate in the treatment of convulsive seizures: toxic symptoms and their prevention. *Arch Neurol Psychiatry* 1939; **42**:1053–1058.
13. **Merritt HH, Putnam TJ.** Sodium diphenyl hydantoinate in the treatment of convulsive seizures: toxic symptoms and their prevention. *Trans Am Neurol Assoc* 1938; **65**:158–162.
14. **Merritt HH, Putnam TJ.** Further experiences with the use of sodium diphenyl hydantoinate in the treatment of convulsive disorders. *Am J Psychiatry* 1940; **96**:1023–1027.
15. **Merritt H, Putnam TJ.** Experimental determination of anticonvulsive activity of chemical compounds. *Epilepsia* 1945; **5**:51–75.
16. **Shorvon SD.** Drug treatment of epilepsy in the century of the ILAE: the second 50 years, 1959–2009. *Epilepsia* 2009; **50**(Suppl 3):93–130.

17. **Bird CAK, Griffen BP, Miklazewska J, Galbraith AW.** Tegretol carbamazepine): a controlled trial of a new anticonvulsant. *Br J Psychiatry* 1966; **112**:737–742.
18. **Meunier H, Carraz G, Meunier Y, Eymard P, Aimard M.** Propriétés pharmacodynamiques de l'acide n-dipropylacétique. [Pharmacodynamic properties of N-dipropylacetic acid]. *Thérapie* 1963; **18**:435–438.
19. **Carraz G, Fau R, Chateau R, Bonnin J.** Communication à propos des premiere essays cliniques sur l'activité anti-épileptique de l'acide n-dipropylacétique (Sel de Na). [Communication concerning first clinical tests of the anticonvulsive activity of N-dipropylacetic acid (sodium salt)]. *Annales médico-psychologiques* 1964; **122**:577–585.
20. **Sternbach L.** The benzodiazepine story. In: Priest RG, Vianna Filho U, Amrein R, Skreta M (eds) *Benzodiazepines Today and Tomorrow*. Lancaster: MTP Press; 1980:5–19.
21. **Shepherd GM.** *Creating Modern Neuroscience*. Oxford: Oxford University Press; 2010.

Chapter 4

Modern Blockbusters

In Chapter 3, we outlined the history of antiepileptic drug development from the 1860s to the 1960s. This coincided with the rise of the pharmaceutical industry into a dominant position both scientifically and commercially, and we now consider what happened next. We ask, too, what has improved since the 1960s, and in fact just how good are our current drugs anyway?

Providing drugs for treatment of epilepsy has proved a multibillion dollar business. Five antiepileptic drugs have reached the fabled blockbuster status (>$1 billion sales per year), albeit for treatment of not only epilepsy but for other central nervous system (CNS) disorders too. These five are levetiracetam (treatment of epilepsy only) which, for example, had peak sales of €1266 million in 2008 but sales figures have been eroded since expiry of patent, lamotrigine (epilepsy and bipolar disorder), topiramate (epilepsy and migraine), gabapentin (epilepsy and neuropathic pain), and pregabalin (epilepsy and neuropathic pain) (1).[1] These drugs generated huge profits and patients and society have paid very large sums for them, and we ask, too, whether the returns for so much money spent have been truly justified.

The Professional Organisations Get Involved

It is probably true to say that it was only in the post-war years that neurologists and others in medical circles began to organise specialised meetings focused on drug therapy. These initiatives were fuelled by sponsorship from the pharmaceutical industry, who to some extent called the tune. Science, medicine, and industry entered a new level of relationship which has caused some unease ever since, but which equally has advanced knowledge and has provided forums for doctors to influence industry.

The Workshops on Neurotransmitters in Epilepsy (WONIEP) are good examples of this, the first being held in Domaine de Seillac, Onzain, France, May 1981 with Paolo Morselli and Kenneth Lloyd of France as organisers (2).

This meeting was in response to the new 'rational' target-based strategies for developing antiepileptic drugs which had emerged in the 1980s. The concept was to identify new antiepileptic drugs based on presumed mechanisms of seizure generation, notably impaired GABAergic inhibition and increased glutamatergic excitation, resulting in antiepileptic drugs that either potentiate GABA transmission (such as vigabatrin and tiagabine) or inhibit glutamate receptors (such as perampanel) (1) (Figure 4.1).

The first workshop was sponsored by Synthélabo, a French drug company that had developed an antiepileptic GABAergic drug called progabide, and not surprisingly, the meeting primarily discussed the role of GABA in epilepsy. At the end of this workshop it was decided to include other neurotransmitters in future meetings, and Ruggero Fariello arranged WONIEP II in San Antonio, Texas, in 1983, which included discussions on catecholamines, opioids, excitatory amino acids, and neuropeptides. At WONIEP III, organised in Soverato, Italy, by Giuseppe Nistico, Paolo Morselli, Kenneth Lloyd, Ruggero Fariello, and Jerome Engel Jr., it became apparent that GABA had proconvulsant, as well as anticonvulsant, properties and the clinical trials of progabide had sadly shown that the drug was not better than placebo (3).[1] This was of course a big disappointment for Paolo Morselli, who had told his audience at a festive meeting organised by Synthélabo in Paris, that progabide was his baby, and as a result, Synthélabo's support for WONIEP IV was stopped. WONIEP IV was held in Stresa, Italy in 1992, but the fading of the GABA wave rendered these efforts no longer viable (4,5). The ILAE then stepped in and funded new workshops, renamed WONOEP (Workshops on the Neurobiology of Epilepsy) which changed the focus from neuropharmacology to neurobiology. These have continued, although it could be argued that the reduction of the influence of the pharmaceutical industry has rendered the translational aspects of these workshops much less effective.

In 1992, a new series of academically inspired conferences was introduced which were deliberately designed to bring together physicians and the industry. These became known as the 'Eilat' conferences, organised by Meir Bialer from Jerusalem and René Levy from Seattle, and these have continued with meetings held every other year. The conferences typically last 4 days with at least 1 day dedicated to antiepileptic drugs in early stages of development, and are characterised by really frank discussion on drug development. Summary reports on a range of new antiepileptic drugs in various stages of development have been published after each conference and have been highly influential.

In the late 1960s, the ILAE had become for the first time a body which government and industry listened to in relation to epilepsy therapy. This was partly indicative of the changing social environment and the growth of lobbying, but also of the outstanding quality of the League's leadership, particularly J. Kiffin Penry and Fritz Dreifuss from the United States, who are the two most eminent epileptologists of their time (6,7). Industry also realised that interaction with the ILAE could improve market share, and so helped oil

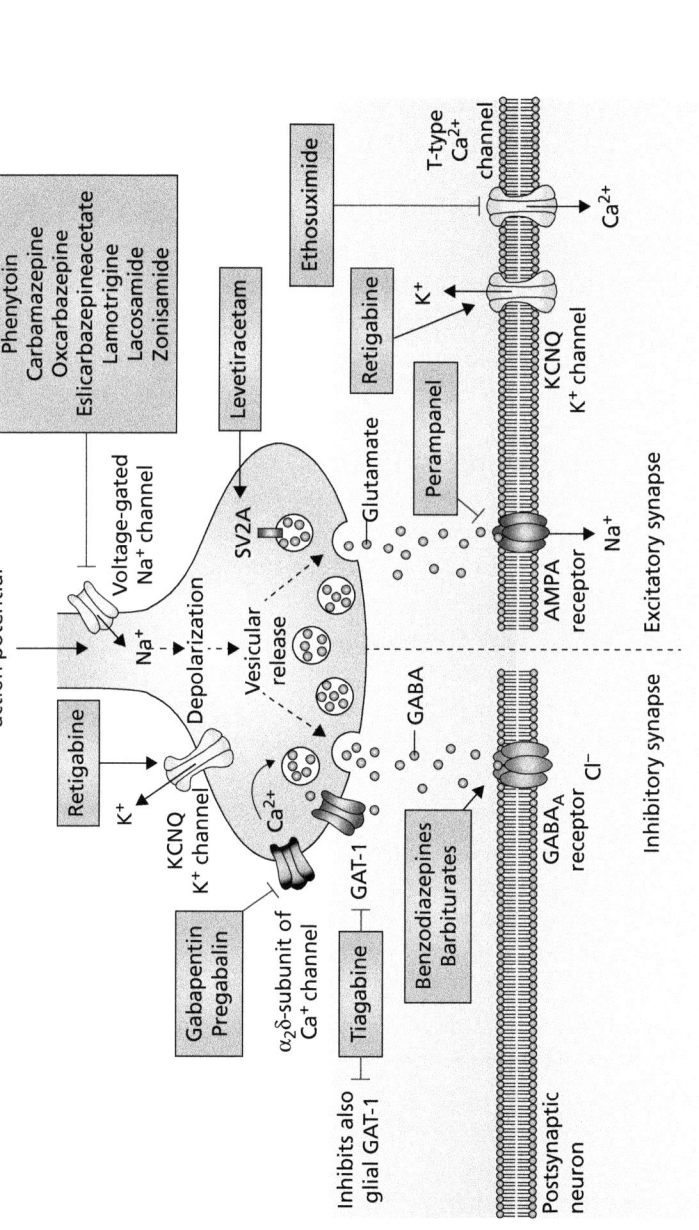

Figure 4.1 Mechanisms of action of antiepileptic drugs, which act by diverse mechanisms, mainly involving modulation of voltage activated ion channels, potentiation of GABA, and inhibition of glutamate (1). Approved antiepileptic drugs have effects on inhibitory (left-hand side) and excitatory (right-hand side) nerve terminals. The antiepileptic efficacy in trials of most of these drugs as initial add-on does not differ greatly, indicating that seemingly similar antiseizure activity can be obtained by mechanisms aimed at diverse targets. However, putative mechanisms of action were determined only after discovering the antiseizure effects; mechanism-driven drug discovery has been largely ignored. AMPA, α-amino-3-hydroxy-5-methyl-4-isoxazole propionic acid; GABA, γ-aminobutyric acid; GAT-1, sodium dependent and chloride dependent GABA transporter 1; SV2A, synaptic vesicle glycoprotein 2A.

Reproduced with permission from Löscher W and Schmidt D, Epilepsy: perampanel—new promise for refractory epilepsy? *Nature Reviews Neurology*, Volume 8, pp. 661–2, Copyright © 2012 Macmillan Publishers Limited.

the wheels of the organisation. Two League activities are of particular note. The ILAE Commission on Antiepileptic Drugs was one of the first ILAE commissions to be established (only the Commission on Classification and Terminology is older) and, it can be argued, its most important. The first meeting, in Scottsville, Arizona, in 1971, was held in close collaboration with the Epilepsy Branch of the National Institute of Neurological Disorders and Stroke (NINDS), a collaboration which proved to be very influential in the 1970s and 1980s. The conference resulted in the publication of the first edition of the book *Antiepileptic Drugs* (now in its fifth edition). In 1973, the commission also published, with the NINDS, a set of influential guidelines for the clinical testing of antiepileptic drugs which were incorporated into the FDA regulations for drug development. The Commission occupied a pre-eminent position in the ILAE, no doubt largely due to the extraordinary energy of its Chairman J. Kiffin Penry. The commissions were constituted for 4-year terms, and the later commissions were less influential than the first. Lennart Gram (8), chair of the Sixth Commission, wrote bitterly to the executive that he could not get any of the commission members to come up with ideas or be active in any way. In 1997, the commission was disbanded and incorporated into a new ILAE Commission on Therapeutic Strategies.

A second notable ILAE initiative was a series of workshops stimulated in the 1970s by the introduction of methods of measuring blood concentrations of antiepileptic drugs, a technology which became known as therapeutic drug monitoring or TDM. Although one of the first studies on the clinical pharmacology of the antiepileptic drug bromide was published as early as 1940 (9), antiepileptic drug monitoring became routine practice only in the 1970s. The workshops were known as the Workshops on the Determination of Antiepileptic Drugs in Body Fluids (under the rather clumsy but memorable acronym WODADIBOF). Between 1972 and 1979, four WODADIBOFs took place, the first in Noordwijkerhout (Netherlands) in April 1972. The second conference took place in Bethel, Germany in 1974 (10). At these, clinical pharmacologists and clinicians discussed the methodologies and value of therapeutic drug monitoring. The workshops also helped promote the quality control schemes for antiepileptic drug measurements first set up by Alan Richens in London.

At ILAE conferences too, pharmacology and drug therapy began to appear, some believe rather belated, in the plenary sessions—and indeed a drug therapy plenary has been incorporated, in some form, in all the International Congresses of the ILAE since 1973, and pharma-sponsored satellites in every conference since 1982.

In 2001, Wolfgang Löscher and Dieter Schmidt from Germany started a series of workshops called New Horizons which took place in Philadelphia

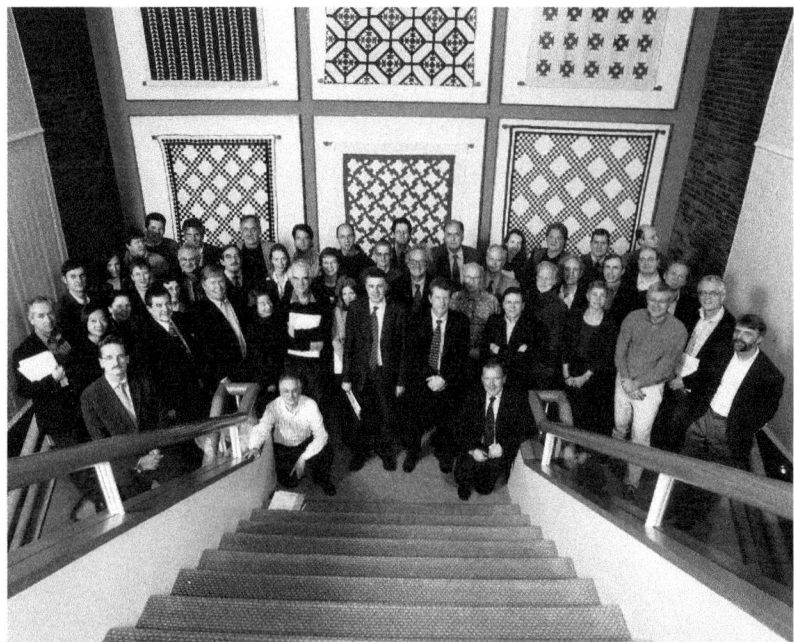

Figure 4.2 The participants of the New Horizons meeting 2003 in Cambridge. Massachusetts, USA which was organised by Wolfgang Löscher and Dieter Schmidt. Reprinted from *Epilepsy Research*, Volume 60, Löscher W and Schmidt D, Conference review: New horizons in the development of antiepileptic drugs: the search for new targets, pp. 77–159, Copyright © 2004 with permission from Elsevier.

in 2001, in Cambridge (United States) in 2003, in Washington, DC in 2005, and in Dublin in 2008 (Figure 4.2 and 4.3) (11). The rationale of the four meetings was the dire fact that despite the development of various novel antiepileptic drugs, about one in five patients with epilepsy is resistant to current pharmacotherapies and furthermore there were no currently available drugs which prevent the development of epilepsy. The meetings thus identified three important goals for the future: (i) better understanding of processes leading to epilepsy, thus allowing the creation of therapies aimed at the prevention of epilepsy in patients at risk; (ii) improved understanding of biological mechanisms of pharmacoresistance, allowing the development of drugs for reversal or prevention of resistance; and (iii) development of disease-modifying therapies, inhibiting the progression of epilepsy. The ultimate goal would be a drug combining these three properties, thus resulting in a complete cure for epilepsy. The New Horizons workshops were very successful in bringing together eminent experimental and clinical scientists to bridge the gap between industry and academia.

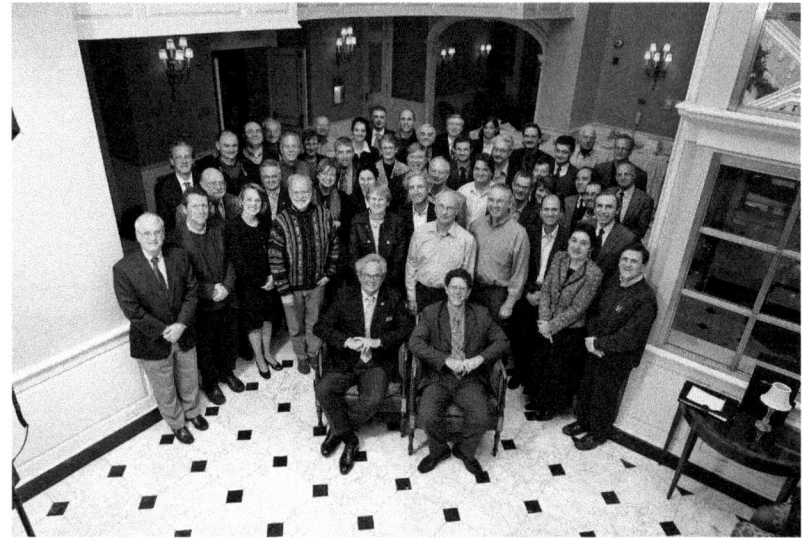

Figure 4.3 New Horizons III in Washington, DC. The third Workshop on New Horizons in the Development of Antiepileptic Drugs explored these four goals for improved epilepsy therapy, with a focus on innovative strategies in the search for better anti-ictal drugs, for novel drugs for prevention of epilepsy or its progression, and for drugs overcoming drug resistance in epilepsy. The current status of antiepileptic therapies under development was critically assessed, and innovative approaches for future therapies are highlighted. The conference review was published (11).
Reprinted from *Epilepsy Research*, Volume 69, Löscher W and Schmidt D, Conference review: New horizons in the development of antiepileptic drugs: Innovative strategies, pp. 183–272, Copyright © 2006 with permission from Elsevier.

The Modern Blockbuster Antiepileptic Drugs

Five antiepileptic drugs marketed in the past 20 years have become winners by industry standards, generating sales of at least US $1 billion per year. However, others that were introduced into the market failed, and many did not even make it to the stage of licensing. It is customary to divide the armamentarium of currently licensed antiepileptic drugs into three groups: first-generation drugs such as phenobarbital and phenytoin; second-generation drugs including carbamazepine, valproate, and benzodiazepines; and third-generation drugs which have been licensed in the last 20 years (12) (Figure 4.4).

The five blockbusters—levetiracetam, lamotrigine, topiramate, gabapentin, and pregabalin—are an interesting study of the interaction of chance, science, and finance; and one thing is quite clear, and that is that luck plays as much as part in drug development as any other factor.

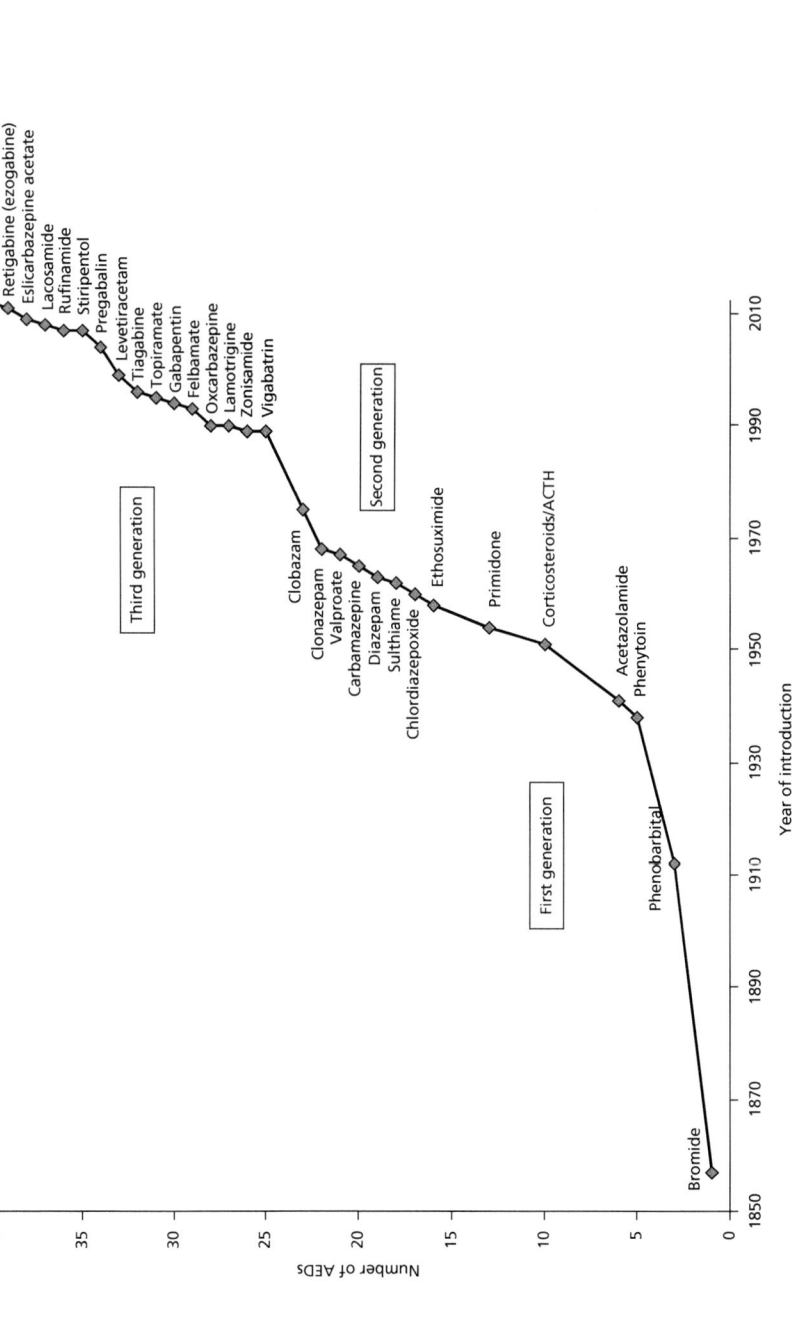

Figure 4.4 Historically, antiepileptic drugs can be classified into three generations. The first generation, entering the market from 1857 to 1958, includes potassium bromide, phenobarbital (PB), and a variety of drugs that were derived mainly by modification of the barbiturate structure, including phenytoin (PHT), primidone (PRM), trimethadione, and ethosuximide (ESM). The second-generation antiepileptic drugs, including carbamazepine (CBZ), valproate (VPA), and the benzodiazepines, which were introduced between 1960 and 1975, differed chemically from the barbiturates. The era of the third-generation antiepileptic drugs started in the 1980s with 'rational' developments such as progabide, vigabatrin (VGB), and tiagabine (TGB), that is, drugs that were designed to selectively target a mechanism that was thought to be critical for the occurrence of epileptic seizures. Reproduced with permission from Löscher W and Schmidt D, Modern antiepileptic drug development has failed to deliver: ways out of the current dilemma. *Epilepsia*, Volume 52, pp. 657–78, Copyright © 2011 John Wiley and Sons, Ltd.

In 1999, levetiracetam entered the market in the United States for treatment of focal-onset seizures of any type in adults. Its antiepileptic drug action had been discovered 7 years earlier, in 1992, by random screening of analogues of piracetam for anticonvulsant effects by Alma J. Gower. She was a scientist working for UCB, at the time a small company which was mostly in the business of making and selling chemicals. Piracetam was one of its few pharmaceuticals, marketed by UCB since the 1950s, a niche drug used by neurologists for many years as an adjunctive drug against cortical myoclonus of any type. Piracetam belongs to a family of cognition-enhancing medicines called nootropics. It was and still is taken by people hoping that it would improve their forgetfulness and possibly preserve their ability to think, especially in South America and in low-income Asian countries, and a Brazilian colleague told us recently that it was widely taken by fellow students at exam times when he was in medical school in the 1980s. The apparent benefits on cognition are likely to have been a therapeutic illusion possibly through a placebo effect, as despite this widespread usage, there is no solid scientific evidence of any cognitive-enhancing effect, and the drug was never licensed for this use in the United Kingdom or United States. In view of the disappointing science, and perhaps because its patent had long run out, UCB embarked on a programme of chemically modifying the structure of piracetam in the hope of finding a better treatment for dementia. In doing so, levetiracetam was created, and by chance therefore what was to become the first blockbuster in epilepsy was born. At the time, UCB did not market any drug for epilepsy, and nobody at UCB expected to discover a blockbuster drug for the treatment of epilepsy, and indeed there was very little initial interest in the drug at the company. Levetiracetam went through the traditional phase I and II stages of evaluation as a cognitive enhancer, and much to the disappointment of UCB it seemed to be as ineffective as piracetam. All new drugs were routinely screened in standard models for anticonvulsant effects, largely to exclude adverse proconvulsant (seizure provoking) activity. Alma J. Gower did her experiments in an audiogenic mice model and discovered that surprisingly the drug had potential anticonvulsant properties. This model was not commonly used to test for antiseizure effects of new compounds, and when tested in the usual gold standard models, the maximal electric shock (MES) and the pentylenetetrazole (PTZ) test where seizures are provoked in rodents by infusion of PTZ, a chemoconvulsant, it had only very weak action. By any industry standards at the time this would have been the end for levetiracetam.

It is an interesting wrinkle to the story how levetiracetam survived and became a blockbuster drug for epilepsy. Before Alma J. Gower submitted her publication she visited the pharmacologist Wolfgang Löscher in Hannover and discussed her findings with him. Löscher became interested in this curious compound and carried out further tests. He discovered that levetiracetam was effective in blocking seizures induced by electrical kindling, a more demanding animal test of epilepsy. His discoveries, and those of Gower, persuaded UCB that they may have a new and unique antiepileptic drug in their hands and they went ahead with costly clinical studies. This is why, with some justification, some people in UCB went so far as to call Wolfgang Löscher the 'godfather of levetiracetam'.[2] It was thus discovered by random screening to see if it was proconvulsant, a classic example of discovery by pure luck (also called serendipity). Ironically, the discovery of levetiracetam, the first blockbuster drug in epilepsy and celebrated as a product of the 'molecular age', was actually not the straightforward innovation by prescient scientists working at the bench in pristine white coats, as romantic minds like to see.

Evidence of how levetiracetam works to stop seizures, in other words its 'mechanism of action', was first reported years later, in 1995, when Noyer and colleagues discovered a stereoselective and brain-specific binding site for levetiracetam and Henrik Klitgaard, a pharmacologist at UCB, and his team then showed that this binding site played an important role in the anticonvulsant properties of levetiracetam (the levetiracetam binding site, LBS). The binding site was considered to reflect a truly unique mechanism for an antiepileptic drug and triggered a cumbersome search for the molecular nature of this binding site, efforts that were rewarded 10 years later when it was discovered that the molecular correlate of the levetiracetam binding site was the synaptic vesicle protein 2A (see Figure 4.1). UCB then initiated a drug-discovery programme searching for ligands with significant affinity to binding site. Variations of the structure of piracetam were systematically studied (the pyrrolidone acetamide scaffold) and this led to the led to the discovery of two further antiepileptic compounds, brivaracetam and seletracetam, with higher affinity and selectivity for this binding site than levetiracetam, and the selection of brivaracetam (13)[3] as the most interesting candidate for further development. It was found to be approximately ten times more potent than levetiracetam as an antiseizure agent in audiogenic seizure-prone mice (14) and a subsequent clinical development programme was performed in over 3000 adult patients which has resulted in licensing of this drug in 2016.

It is worth noting that although both brivaracetam and seletracetam were identified years ago, their release onto the market was dictated partly by commercial considerations. It was decided not to do so until the patent of levetiracetam had run out, and obviously the two drugs were competitors for each other, a situation which although would have assisted clinical practice clearly made no commercial sense. The problem now is how to overcome the hurdle of trying to show that the two are different drugs and that both are better than levetiracetam. Generic manufacture of levetiracetam, which is an extremely popular antiepileptic drug, is widespread and marketing is focusing on brivaracetam. Both seem to rather similar compounds and marketing may have to shoulder the burden of differentiation that science could not yet achieve.

Despite the commercial success of levetiracetam, no randomised blinded controlled study has shown it to be any more effective than older standard antiepileptic drugs such as carbamazepine or valproate for the treatment of focal or generalised seizures although it may be less sedative and causes fewer hypersensitivity reactions than carbamazepine and is certainly less teratogenic than valproate. It is easier to use than the other drugs, due to the absence of hypersensitivity reactions and bothersome drug interactions, but do these medical advantages alone explain the commercial success of levetiracetam? Probably not. The company was also very skilful in marketing and succeeded in selling levetiracetam at a much higher price than comparable older drugs for epilepsy. Furthermore, levetiracetam was launched into the market at a time when regulatory agencies were only interested in evidence that the drug is effective and safe. Nobody required evidence that it was better than available treatment to justify the higher price. It was probably the juste milieu of good medicine, an exciting new mechanism of action, bold marketing, and relaxed attention to the cost that made levetiracetam the only blockbuster among drugs used for epilepsy alone.

The tremendous commercial success of drugs such as levetiracetam prompts the question of why do physicians prefer one among many other agents with very similar medical properties when looking at the risk:benefit balance of each compound with a cold eye? We like to believe that prescribing a new drug is based entirely on a rational assessment of the scientific pros and cons of the agent. However, recent research has uncovered that other factors may be just as important. Suggestions by pharmaceutical representatives, observation of hospital prescribing, and patients' requests for a specific drug may play an important role (15). Marketing efforts using recent insights from neuro-economics that aim to appeal to the brain's reward system may possibly better explain why new antiepileptic drugs are preferred which seem to offer no substantial medical benefits in efficacy over older drugs.

Although it is difficult in general, to quantify, the contribution of marketing to the success of a drug, the marketing itself has become very sophisticated, and one example is the use of what is known as integrated segmentation (16). In this method, the individual doctor's personal attitudes, values and 'psychographies' are explored and categorised by the pharmaceutical company representatives who then use this information to plan a suitably targeted approach to its physician customers (16). A final wrinkle to the story of levetiracetam is that its main side effect, a change in behaviour causing irritability, anger, 'short fuse', and dysphoric mood was not noted at all in the clinical trials—showing one common lesson of antiepileptic drug studies, that within the straitjacket of a clinical trial, important effects can be missed and it is important to maintain strict observation of all new drugs even after licensing and try to see through the blue haze of the marketing slogans. Finally, strangely, many patients who develop irritability or dysphoria while taking levetiracetam rarely attribute this to levetiracetam but often blame themselves or stressful personal interactions, in striking contrast to the more common tendency to blame a drug for everything. Levetiracetam is also exceptional in that, unlike all other blockbuster drugs for epilepsy, it has no important sales outside its use in epilepsy. All in all, levetiracetam is a remarkable modern, easy-to-use, and reasonably well tolerated standard antiepileptic drug that has brought seizure relief to many patients. Physicians and patients alike are happy to have it at their disposal, which is no small feat for any drug.

In 1990, lamotrigine was approved in Europe, and in 1994 in the United States, as an adjunctive therapy for focal epilepsy in adult patients, and has since become a standard monotherapy treatment for focal seizures and adjunctive therapy for absence seizures and myoclonic seizures. From the commercial view, though, it was also the finding that it lowers the risk of episodes in patients with bipolar disorder and proves, like valproate, to be a mood stabiliser (which can be also beneficial for epilepsy patients) that has delivered the most profit and elevated the drug to the status of blockbuster.

The story of its discovery, like that of levetiracetam, is no tale of rational scientific development, but one of faulty theory, astute clinical observation, and a large dose of luck. Lamotrigine was synthesised in the early 1980s on the premise that antifolate compounds would be good antiepileptic drugs. This was based on evidence dating from the mid-1960's that folate was proconvulsant and the knowledge that phenobarbital and phenytoin in use at the time were folic acid antagonists, The folate theory was proposed in 1966 by the well-known London epileptologist Dr Edward ('Ted') Reynolds, and the British pharmaceutical company Burroughs-Wellcome became interested as they already had marketed the antifolate compound pyrimethamine for the treatment of malaria.

Burroughs-Wellcome modified the molecule of pyrimethamine and among the series of compounds developed, lamotrigine was found to have considerable anticonvulsant activity in routine animal testing. This effect though has nothing to do with any antifolate action and as it has turned out, lamotrigine is in fact only a weak inhibitor of dihydrofolate reductase, and stronger antifolate drugs, such as methotrexate, which were also produced by Burroughs-Wellcome, did not have anticonvulsant properties. It has subsequently become clear that lamotrigine owes its antiepileptic activity to sodium channel inhibition, and not to its weak antifolate effect. A prime example of a chance discovery based on a wrong hypothesis.

Drs Anthony ('Tony') W. Peck and Alan Yuen were clinical investigators at GlaxoSmithKline, the pharmaceutical company that eventually marketed the blockbuster lamotrigine, and they have nicely described the discovery process (17). Lamotrigine first entered human phase I studies in healthy volunteers in the early 1980s and an extensive series of often small clinical trials culminated in its first approval for use in epilepsy in 1990 in Ireland, followed by worldwide regulatory approvals for epilepsy over the next several years.

An unexpected puzzle emerged in these early studies when the epilepsy trial reports were returned to the company. Curiously, patients opted to continue lamotrigine in extension studies though their diaries did not show improved seizure counts. Some patients receiving lamotrigine treatment reported improved mood and noted that they were more communicative and agreeable, reminiscent of earlier observations with valproate and carbamazepine, which had originally led to the suggestion that antiepileptic drugs might be useful in the treatment of bipolar disorder. Robert Post and colleagues at the National Institute of Mental Health (NIMH) hypothesised that an overactive limbic system was involved in mood swings, leading to the search for, and testing of therapeutic agents like carbamazepine that were effective in animal tests perceived as models of limbic epilepsy. Because of this, a full clinical development programme was started and lamotrigine is today a standard drug for bipolar disease. Finally, it is noteworthy that despite the commercial success, like levetiracetam, lamotrigine has never been shown to be more effective than older antiepileptic drugs such as carbamazepine for the treatment of focal seizures, and this is a topic to which we return later.

Topiramate is another blockbuster with antiepileptic effects discovered by chance, this time in a project seeking a new antidiabetic agent. It was originally synthesised in research to discover structural analogues of fructose-1,6-diphosphate capable of inhibiting the enzyme fructose-1,6-diphosphatase which blocks gluconeogenesis and thus might work in diabetes mellitus. Topiramate is a derivative of a naturally occurring monosaccharide D-fructose and contains a sulphamate moiety and was prepared as a synthetic intermediate in the project. Disappointingly, topiramate turned out to have no hypoglycaemic activity and thus was ineffective in the treatment of diabetes mellitus. However, when routinely tested for anti- or proconvulsant activity, topiramate was found to be highly active in the traditional maximal electroshock seizure test in mice and rats, and possessed a particularly long duration of action. Furthermore, there was a wide separation between the effective anticonvulsant doses compared to those causing motor side effects. Subsequent studies indicated effects of topiramate on several protein complexes including voltage-gated sodium channels, $GABA_A$ receptors, and AMPA/kainite receptors (see Figure 4.1). It then entered clinical trials in epilepsy and was found to be highly efficacious. The main problems of topiramate in epilepsy are related to a high rate of side effects. This was despite the apparently good preclinical performance in healthy rodents in this regard demonstrating again the loose correlation between clinical and preclinical findings. The reputation for side effects derived initially from a memorable presentation made at the topiramate satellite symposium at the Oslo International Epilepsy Congress in 1993, where one speaker showed a slide of a single patient with 13 different side effects and thenceforward the engrained reputation proved hard to shake off. The great efficacy of the drug though has never been in doubt and in the famous meta-analysis of antiepileptic trials reported in 1997, topiramate was found to be the drug with the greatest antiepileptic effect (18).

The positive effect of topiramate in migraine was also discovered serendipitously. In the early years after its launch, several physicians noted the antimigraine effect in their patients and reported this to Joe Hulihan who was employed by the medical affairs organisation of Johnson & Johnson at the time. He approached academic migraine physicians to discuss the observations and the potential to develop topiramate in the migraine indication (prevention/prophylaxis). Johnson & Johnson did a meta-analysis in two very small investigator-initiated studies, confirmed the integrity of the datasets, and proceeded with a combined dose finding and confirmatory phase II/III programme. So the pathway was from practitioners, to the company, and then to the headache specialist community for input, building internal confidence in the signal, and then a decision to a rather bold jump into a new indication (Roy Twyman, personal communication). It is the migraine indication, not the epilepsy one, which has resulted in its blockbuster status.

Gabapentin, and the structurally related pregabalin, are blockbuster antiepileptic drugs which, as it has turned out, have much great utility in the treatment of pain. Gabapentin entered the US market in 1993 for adjunctive treatment of focal seizures in adults but curiously is not approved for marketing as monotherapy in the United States. The drug was discovered by chance by a chemist working for Gödecke AG in Freiburg, Germany. Gerhard Satzinger tried to improve the oral bioavailability of GABA through the incorporation of lipophilic groups on the carbon backbone. Although compounds described in Satzinger's original work did possess anticonvulsant activity (as did centrally administered

GABA), it was ultimately found that none of these compounds affected either metabotropic or ionotropic GABA receptors, nor fluxed through the blood–brain barrier by passive diffusion. However, it was from these fortuitous studies that gabapentin emerged as an efficacious anticonvulsant in routine screening with the less often used thiosemicarbazide-induced tonic convulsion model in mice. Several years later, its anticonvulsant properties were confirmed in the low-intensity mouse electroshock test.

Clinical phase II studies with gabapentin began in 1983 and continued in 1984 and 1985 with several quite small studies against Huntington's disease, hemiplegia, and spasticity (single-blind and placebo-controlled) and not epilepsy. Gabapentin was initially evaluated as an antispastic compound because of its structural similarity to baclofen and its ability to attenuate the polysynaptic spinal reflex in animal models of spasticity. The antispastic effects of gabapentin proved to be modest. This trial offers an interesting insight into how an important discovery can be missed. Case report forms of spasticity trials in the Netherlands and Spain were largely negative. However, nearly all patients reported to have less pain when taking gabapentin. At the time, the company attributed that to the anti-spasticity effect of the compound, and an opportunity to discover the effect of gabapentin on pain at an early stage was lost. Gabapentin has since become a blockbuster pain medication, and one that has only limited use in epilepsy (19).[4]

The first clinical study of gabapentin in epilepsy showing efficacy was conducted with 25 patients in 1985 as a placebo-controlled add-on crossover study in refractory partial seizures and there was a marked response (20). A clinical development programme was launched by a planning team at first chaired by Bernd Schmidt, a neurologist, and run from Gödecke in Freiburg situated close to the Black Forest in Germany. When Gödecke was bought by Pfizer, the clinical development was continued, it has been said, with some reservations for two reasons: (i) Pfizer had bought a licence for zonisamide, an antiepileptic drug on the market in Japan and (ii) because of 'NIH = not invented here', and some researchers at Pfizer referred to it as the Black Forest drug and were said to show little interest in it (Bernd Schmidt, personal communication). The road that gabapentin took at Pfizer was tortuous and its development was close to being terminated by the Pfizer management three times during the development according to Bernd Schmidt. This is an example that drug development is never as straightforward, linear, and rational as we often like to believe. In January 1995, two pain specialists, Larry B. Mellick from Loma Linda, California, and Gary A. Mellick from Lorain, Ohio, sent a letter to the *American Journal of Emergency Medicine* (21) reporting that gabapentin, a newly released anticonvulsant, unexpectedly worked very well in five patients with reflex sympathetic dystrophy. This clinical observation seems to have been the first published report that gabapentin had an effect on pain, and led to this turning out to be a black swan product (22)[5] with a commercial impact that has dwarfed the success of its antiseizure effect.

This brings us finally to the discovery of pregabalin, a close structural relation of gabapentin, and a drug which evolved in rather different circumstances. It was discovered by Richard Silverman, a university chemist, and became a blockbuster drug that has showered him and Northwestern University with more than $700 million in royalties. There was an interesting article in the *Chicago Tribune* in 2008 from Silverman in which he describes how his drug was whisked away behind the curtain of big pharma not to be seen or heard about for many years. Apparently when he expressed an interest in attending the launch party, he was told no.

Pregabalin is a rare example of a compound that came straight out of academia to become a commercially viable drug (22), and how it was discovered is a fascinating story. The drug is a very close analogue of the neurotransmitter GABA. Silverman's lab made a series of compounds in the 1980s to try to inhibit the aminotransferase enzyme (GABA-AT) that breaks GABA down in the brain, as a means of increasing its levels to prevent epileptic seizures. They gradually realised, though, that their compounds were also activating another enzyme, glutamic acid decarboxylase (GAD), which actually synthesises GABA. Shutting down the neurotransmitter's breakdown was a good idea, but shutting down its production at the same time clearly wasn't going to work. So in 1988, a visiting Polish post-doc, Ryszard Andruszkiewicz, made a series of 3-alkyl GABA and glutamate analogues in an attempt to find a more selective compound. Northwestern University, on the basis of this profile, offered the compounds to industry, and Parke-Davis took them up. One enantiomer of the 3-isobutyl GABA analogue turned out to be a star performer in the company's rodent assay for antiseizure effect, and attempts to find an even better compound were fruitless. The next few years were spent on toxicity testing and optimising the synthetic route. The Investigational New Drug paperwork to use this analogue in humans was filed in 1995, and clinical trials continued until 2003. The FDA approved the drug in 2004. This is not an unusual timeline for drug development, especially for a CNS compound. And there you might think the story ends—basic science from the university is translated into a big-selling drug, with the unusual feature of an actual compound from the academic labs going all the way.

But, as Silverman makes clear, there's a lot more to the story. As it turned out, the drug's efficacy had nothing to do with its GABA-AT substrate behaviour. Further investigation showed that it has no action on the other enzyme,

GAD. In other words, despite its effectiveness in animal testing, neither of the actions underpinning the compound's sale to Parke-Davis held up. The biologists at Parke-Davis eventually discovered that the compound also binds to a particular site on voltage-gated calcium channels, and that it blocks the release of glutamate, whose actions would be opposed to those of GABA. Better still, Parke-Davis found out that the compound was taken up by active transport into the brain which also helps account for its strong activity, and because of its smaller dosage and stronger binding, unlike gabapentin, pregabalin has a more favourable linear uptake profile without transporter saturation at therapeutic dosages. Silverman goes on to show that while the compound was originally designed as a GABA analogue, it doesn't have any action at the GABA receptor and doesn't affect GABA levels in any way. It seems that a thorough, careful pharmacological analysis before going into animals would probably have killed the compound before it was even tested, which goes to show how important animal data are even when we don't understand yet how the drug works. It also shows that knowing the mechanism is not essential for finding a good drug.

So, on one level, this is indeed an academic compound that went to industry and became a drug. But looked at from another perspective, it was an extremely lucky shot indeed, for several unrelated reasons, and the underlying biology was only worked out once the compound went into industrial development. And from any angle, it's an object lesson in how little we know, and how many surprises are waiting for us. As a footnote, it is worth recording that a true inhibitor of GABA-AT was discovered in Strasbourg, France, a drug called vigabatrin. This proved to have strong antiseizure action and was marked for epilepsy in quite a few countries, but turned out to cause visual failure due to retinal toxicity and due to this side effect has been effectively withdrawn from almost all practice, at least in adult-onset epilepsy.

Is industry losing interest in epilepsy?

During the past three decades, the introduction of 17 new antiepileptic drugs has provided physicians and patients with more options for the treatment of many types of seizures. For rare epilepsies, new additive drugs such as stiripentol have brought better seizure control in some patients, but for most types of epilepsy there is no evidence of dramatically better effectiveness of the newer drugs when compared to the (much cheaper) older compounds. The fact that antiepileptic drugs provide relief from seizures in over 80% of patients in the long term means that epilepsy is one of the most treatable of all neurological conditions, with a success rate that is much higher than in stroke, Parkinson's disease, dementia, or brain tumour for instance. That the older drugs are so efficacious is creating a problem for the pharmaceutical industry developing new drugs as the new compounds have to be shown to be somehow better than the already good old agents.

Because of the lack of striking differentiation in terms of efficacy, the industry turned to a new battlefield in an effort to promote its new medicines—and that was the issue of side effects. Drug side effects occur in every second patient starting an antiepileptic drug. Most side effects are neurological and mild but occasionally antiepileptic drugs may have fatal side effects. These can be either directly life-threatening or indirectly so by increasing the risk for life-threatening depression or aggression. The most vulnerable are patients, unkindly referred as double-losers, who continue to have seizures and usually receive higher daily doses or several drugs which increases side effects. Although there have been strenuous efforts by the marketing departments of pharmaceutical companies to persuade physicians to the contrary, the fact remains that as a group, the newer drugs have a generally similar range of side effects as the older drugs. This, with similar efficacy, is a disappointment. Even worse than this is the fact that it was a problem with side effects too which dictated the removal of some new drugs from routine practice, resulting in multimillion dollar failures; these included the hepatic failure and aplastic anaemia which sealed the fate of felbamate, the visual field defects of vigabatrin, and the pigmentary changes in skin, nails, and retina due to retigabine.

From an industry perspective it seems that until the 1990s, epilepsy presented an opportunity which offered a good chance for high returns on investment. There was an unmet need with few treatment options (especially for patients with refractory seizures), few competitors, as well as manageable technical and regulatory hurdles. The adjunctive or add-on treatment trial design for refractory epilepsy propelled large numbers of new antiepileptic drugs to the market. The placebo-controlled adjunctive trial design for evaluating the efficacy of a test compound in refractory epilepsy established efficacy and tolerability at an early stage and could be performed using cost-efficient, short-term clinical studies lasting a few months. This template provided an incentive for several companies to bring new antiepileptic drugs to the market.

Investment in antiepileptic drug development, however, then met a new hurdle. Prompted by efforts to contain expenditures for health for government, reimbursement required that future antiepileptic drugs bring additional clinical value or differentiation (principally an improvement in efficacy) to an already crowded, highly generic antiepileptic drug field. In addition, differentiation by safety profile for new antiepileptic drugs is not considered a principal component for optimising pricing and reimbursement beyond the tight regulatory control to bring safe products to the market. New regulatory hurdles have also evolved over the past decades. A generally lower risk tolerance for new drugs and recent class labelling regarding safety signals, for instance in relation to suicide or teratogenicity, have affected opportunities in non-epilepsy indications and had an impact on the overall value proposition for antiepileptic drugs. Development of new antiepileptic drugs can require long-term safety data in different age populations, and paediatric investigational plans necessitate the development and testing of new formulations in very young patients (babies who are ≥1 month old). The pharmaceutical companies have decided that an adjunctive epilepsy indication alone is not adequate given the current regulations, and that the cost of approval of a monotherapy licence causes too great a time delay and additional cost. The industry is, it seems, therefore losing interest in developing novel compounds for epilepsy. Taken together with perceptions that better return on investment is more likely in other therapeutic areas, such as multiple sclerosis or Parkinson's disease, this has prompted several major drug companies to leave the field of epilepsy in the search for more profitable developments. Indeed, some of the largest pharmaceutical companies have exited from the whole field of neurology in view of the difficulties of testing and assessment. There is general agreement among specialists that we need now to revitalise the discovery and the development of future antiepileptic drugs (see Chapter 8). What are needed are new paradigms of discovery, new preclinical testing paradigms, and new paradigms for clinical trial—a step change in each is required.

Notes

1. In an early randomised controlled trial, progabide, an experimental GABAergic antiepileptic drug, was given in a placebo-controlled, double-blind cross-over trial to 19 adult patients with chronic partial epilepsy refractory to previous high-dose antiepileptic drug therapy. Progabide did not significantly change the seizure frequency. In patients with a therapeutic response, progabide led to an increase in the plasma concentration of phenytoin and phenobarbital. Co-medication with carbamazepine was associated with a poor response to progabide. Side effects were mild except for a several-fold increase of liver enzymes SGOT and SGPT, which required withdrawal of progabide in one patient. The study authors dryly noted that progabide does not seem to be the drug urgently needed for failures of previous high-dose drug therapy (3).
2. For those interested in nuts and bolts of the discovery: Dr Wolfgang Löscher and his colleague Doris Hönack confirmed that UCB L059 (levetiracetam) was ineffective in the traditional maximal electroshock seizure and subcutaneous PTZ seizure tests in mice and rats even at very high doses of up to 500 mg/kg. They showed that UCB L059 increased the thresholds for tonic electroconvulsions and myoclonic and clonic seizures induced by timed intravenous infusion of pentylenetetrazole (PTZ). The anticonvulsant potency of UCB L059 in seizure threshold tests was, however, surprisingly similar to that of standard drugs, such as valproate. Much to everybody's surprise, UCB L059 exerted

potent anticonvulsant activity against both focal and secondarily generalised seizures in amygdala-kindled rats. These findings were further refined by Henrik Klitgaard, an epilepsy pharmacologist who joined UCB as Head of the Neuroscience Area in 1994, by the demonstration that UCB059 systematically showed selective anticonvulsant activity in animal models of acquired and genetic epilepsy contrasted by an absence of seizure protection against acute seizures in normal animals induced by a maximal electroshock of bolus dose of chemoconvulsants.

3. Its chemical name is (2S)-2-[(4R)-2-oxo-4-propylpyrrolidin-1-yl]butanamide 83alpha (UCB 34714).

4. Very early on, Bernd Schmidt, a neurologist working at Gödecke, drafted the graph with the first development plan that included indications other than epilepsy (Bernd Schmidt, personal communication) (20).

5. Black swan is a term used to designate unusual phenomena that turn out to be highly influential and consequential, and yet were neither predicted nor anticipated (21).

References

1. **Löscher W, Schmidt D.** Epilepsy: perampanel—new promise for refractory epilepsy? *Nat Rev Neurol* 2012; **8**:661–662.
2. **Morselli P, Lloyd KG, Löscher W, Meldrum BS, Reynolds EH** (eds). *Neurotransmitters, Seizures, and Epilepsy*. New York: Raven Press; 1981.
3. **Schmidt D, Utech K.** Progabide for refractory partial epilepsy: a controlled add-on trial. *Neurology* 1986; **36**(2):217–221.
4. **Avanzini G, Engel JJr, Fariello R, Heinemann U** (eds). Neurotransmitters in epilepsy. *Epilepsy Research* 1992; Suppl 8.
5. **Engel JJr, Moshé S, Avanzini G.** Organisation of basic science in epilepsy with special reference to the International League Against Epilepsy. In: Shorvon S, Weiss G, Avanzini G, et al. (eds) *International League Against Epilepsy 1909–2009*. Chichester: Wiley-Blackwell; 2009:143–152.
6. **Dreifuss FE.** J. Kiffin Penry 1929–1996. *Epilepsia* 1996; **37**:1023–1024.
7. **Porter R.** Fritz E. Dreifuss 1926–1997. *Epilepsia* 1998; **39**:556–559.
8. **Alving J, Pedersen B.** Lennart Gram 1948–1999. *Epilepsia* 1999; **49**:1325–1328.
9. **Walker G.** *Measurement of Bromide Levels in Urine, Blood and Cerebrospinal Fluid and their Relevance for Epilepsy Therapy* (in German). Dissertation of the Medical Faculty Zurich University Buchdruck. A. Fausch; 1940.
10. **Schneider H, Janz D, Gardner-Thorpe C, Meinardi H, Sherwin AL** (eds). *Clinical Pharmacology of Anti-Epileptic Drugs. Workshop on the Determination of Anti-Epileptic Drugs in Body Fluid II (WODADIBOF II) Held in Bethel, Bielefeld, Germany, 24–25 May, 1974*. Heidelberg: Springer; 1975.
11. **Löscher W, Schmidt D.** New Horizons in the development of antiepileptic drugs: Innovative strategies. *Epilepsy Res* 2006; **69**:183–272.
12. **Löscher W, Schmidt D.** Modern antiepileptic drug development has failed to deliver: ways out of the current dilemma. *Epilepsia* 2011; **52**:657–678.
13. **Zaccara G, Schmidt D.** Do traditional anti-seizure drugs have a future? A review of potential anti-seizure drugs in clinical development. *Pharmacol Res* 2015; **104**:38–48.

14. **Kenda BM, Matagne AC, Talaga PE,** et al. Discovery of 4-substituted pyrrolidone butanamides as new agents with significant antiepileptic activity. *J Med Chem* 2004; **47**(3):530–549.
15. **Prosser H, Almond S, Walley T.** Influences on GPs' decision to prescribe new drugs- the importance of who says what. *Fam Pract* 2003; **20**(1):61–68.
16. **Brand R, Kumar P.** *Detailing Gets Personal: Integrated Segmentation may be Pharma's Key to 'Repersonalizing' the Selling Process.* PharmExec.com; 1 August 2003. [Online] http://www.pharmexec.com/detailing-gets-personal
17. **Peck AW.** Lamotrigine: historical background. *Rev Contemp Pharmacother* 1994; **5**:95–105.
18. **Marson AG, Kadir ZA, Hutton JL, Chadwick DW.** The new antiepileptic drugs: a systematic review of their efficacy and tolerability. *Epilepsia* 1997; **38**(8):859–880.
19. **Mellick LB, Mellick GA.** Successful treatment of reflex sympathetic dystrophy with gabapentin. *Am J Emerg Med* 1995; **13**:96.
20. **Schmidt B.** Gabapentin. In: Levy R, Mattson R, Meldrum B, Penry JK, Dreifuss FE (eds) *Antiepileptic Drugs,* 3rd ed. New York: Raven Press, Ltd; 1989:925–35.
21. **Taleb N.** *The Black Swan: The Impact of the Highly Improbable.* New York: Random House; 2007.
22. **Silverman RB.** From basic science to blockbuster drug: the discovery of Lyrica. *Angew Chem Int Ed Engl* 2008; **47**(19):3500–3504.

Chapter 5

Resecting Epilepsy

One reason for starting our history in the year 1860 is that it was then that the possibilities for surgical treatment of epilepsy were opening up a new era of therapeutics and new promise for patients with epilepsy—it even seemed possible to some at the time that neurosurgery going to provide a means to end epilepsy, but this has proved wildly over-optimistic.

The Evolution of Surgery for Epilepsy

Neurosurgery had become feasible because of four fundamental scientific developments in this period: antisepsis and asepsis, anaesthesia with chloroform and orotracheal intubation, the discovery that different functions were located in different locations in the brain (a theory known as cerebral localisation), and the realisation that the location of the seizure discharge could be predicted from its symptomatology.

The invention of surgical antisepsis is attributed to (Lord) Joseph Lister who was Professor of Surgery at the University of Glasgow.[1] He read Louis Pasteur's papers on infection by micro-organisms and decided killing them by chemical means would be a possible way of reducing surgical infection. He experimented with various compounds and selected carbolic acid (as its derivative creosote had been used for treating sewerage). His first treatment was in 1865 and he published his results in *The Lancet* in 1867. He instructed surgeons to wear gloves, to wash their hands and instruments in 5% carbolic acid solutions, and to spray the solution in the operating theatre. The results were dramatic, and infection rates plummeted. The carbolic spray, disagreeable as it is to the nose, was to change surgery for ever and to extend its possibilities even to operating on exposed brain tissue, which prior to this was wholly out of bounds.

The use of chloroform for surgical anaesthesia also was first attempted by another Scottish doctor, (Sir) James Young Simpson in 1847, as was orotracheal intubation[2] first used, during chloroform anaesthesia by (Sir) William Macewen in Glasgow in 1878.[3] Sir Victor Horsley, of whom more below, experimented with ether and chloroform in animals, and also on himself, as Simpson had done and nearly died. He then also developed, with the chemist Vernon Harcourt in Oxford, a method of administering 2% of chloroform, in an intubated patient, via a vaporiser connected to a compressed oxygen cylinder. These inventions set the scene for human neurosurgery. The first surgeons to operate on the brain were (Sir) William Macewen in Glasgow in 1877 and (Sir) Rickman Godlee, Lister's nephew, who carried out the first operation on a patient with epilepsy and a cerebral glioma in London in 1884. However, it was Sir Victor Horsley who was the greatest of all these early surgeons and he earns the privilege of being named the 'Father of Neurosurgery'.

The scientific discovery that some brain functions were located in specific parts of the brain (the theory of 'cerebral localisation'), which was indeed one of the landmark medical advances of the nineteenth century, was the basis for epilepsy surgery. Prior to this, the predominant view was that the brain was largely undifferentiated (the theory of equipotentiality) and it was only when researchers began to activate different areas of exposed brain with small electrical currents, a process known as cortical stimulation, that it became apparent that different areas of the brain had different functions. Pioneers in the field were Gustav Fritsch and Eduard Hitzig in Germany and David Ferrier in England. Ferrier carried out extensive comparative studies in a variety of animals, and constructed maps of the functions of different areas of cortex. He identified areas controlling movements and sensation and also vision. Ferrier remarked that his reason for conducting these experiments was to confirm 'the theories about localisation' of his mentor, John Hughlings Jackson, who had in the previous decade made similar predictions about localised brain function based on his clinical observations of patients and the subsequent pathological examinations of their post-mortem brains.

It was Jackson, too, who surmised that, as different forms of epileptic seizure were caused by excessive discharges in different parts of the brain, their symptoms of the seizure could indicate from which part of the brain the seizure arose. As Ferrier put it, by his 'artificial reproduction of the clinical experiments performed by disease' using cortical stimulation. He also confirmed Jackson's theory that epilepsies are caused by discharging cortical lesions.[4]

A famous event in the history of cerebral localisation was the confrontation between Ferrier and Friedrich Leopold Goltz, Professor of Physiology at the University of Strasburg, at the 1881 Seventh International Medical Congress held in London.[5] Goltz was an advocate of equipotentiality and to support his views he demonstrated a live dog which he claimed had been subjected to wide removal of the cerebral cortex but was not paralysed. Ferrier then expounded his own localisationist theories and to prove his point showed a live and hemiplegic monkey which he claimed had 7 months previously had an only small and localised unilateral resection of the motor cortex. Charcot was present and was so impressed by the nature of the hemiplegia in the macaque that he exclaimed 'C'est un malade!'. Ferrier accused Goltz of flawed experimental technique and both offered to allow the brains of the animals to be studied by an independent committee. This was done, and the committee reported back a few days later that Goltz's operation had not removed the central cortical areas as he had asserted, and that the circumscribed lesion in the motor area of Ferrier's monkey was exactly as Ferrier had claimed. Horsley, Godlee, and Macewen were in the audience at the congress, and this event must have been a stimulus to their subsequent forays into neurosurgery.

There was wide publicity of these events, which proved too much for the powerful antivivisectionist movement in England at the time. Shortly after the congress, Ferrier was indicted and summoned to appear in court, accused of performing 'Frightful and shocking experiments'. Horsley, Charcot, Jackson, Lister, and other famous scientists attended the court proceedings, which were widely publicised in the national and international press, and Ferrier was exonerated (albeit on somewhat of a technicality). This added further renown to the theories of cerebral localisation, which then became a focus of intense worldwide scientific research for the next several decades.

Horsley himself was carrying out a series of remarkable experiments in which, by electrical stimulation, he localised function in the brains of macaque monkeys and orangutans and then armed with the knowledge produced a series of elegant and highly sophisticated minute functional maps of the primate cerebral cortex. He based his work on the comparative anatomy of human and primate brains, using the primate experiments to predict the site of onset of human seizures in human patients, on the supposition that the symptoms at the onset of the seizures represented activation of localised regions of brain, as Jackson and Ferrier had suggested.

Observed by Jackson and Ferrier, Horsley proceeded then to carry out a series of surgical operations for epilepsy at the National Hospital for the Paralysed and Epileptic at Queen Square in London (Figure 5.1). His first operation was on 25 May 1886, on a patient with post-traumatic epilepsy, caused 15 years earlier by a depressed fracture of the skull. His seizures started with jerking in the right leg and spread to involve the right arm and face with turning of the head and eyes to the right. Horsley predicted the site of the epileptic focus on the basis of these symptoms and opened the skull and the brain covering over the central cortex of the left hemisphere and found, as he had predicted, a scar from the head injury (Figure 5.2). He excised this and the operation resulted in a complete resolution of seizures. The second patient was operated upon on 26 June 1886, and was perhaps more audacious in the sense that there was no depressed fracture to provide ancillary information about localisation. The patient was a 20-year-old man who had recently developed epilepsy. Horsley

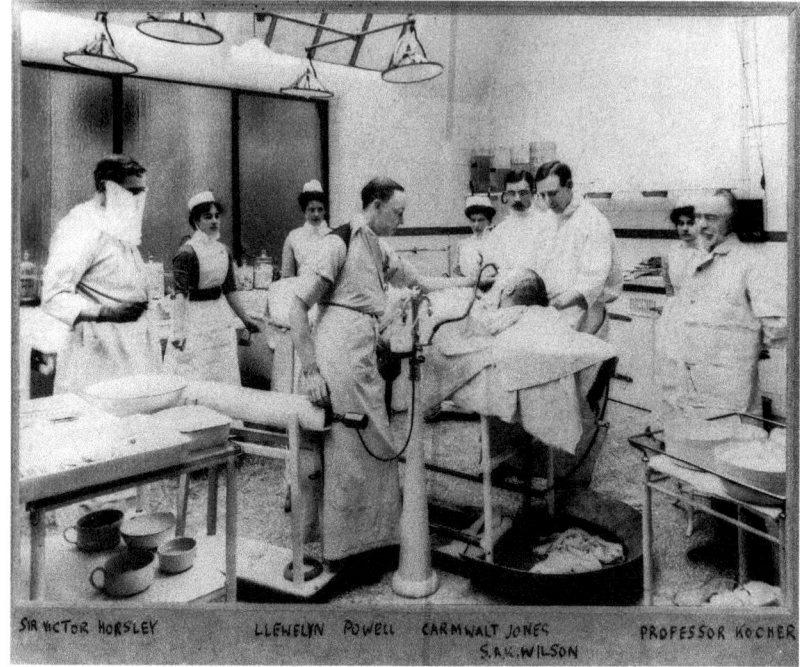

Figure 5.1 This is a famous photograph of Victor Horsley in 1906 in his operating theatre at the National Hospital. Horsley is on the left—gowned and masked. His gown is bulky for underneath were sterile dressings preparing him for an appendicectomy which he had on the next day. Also in the photograph are S. A. K. Wilson, Carmalt Jones, and Emil Kocher a few years before he was awarded the Nobel Prize. The celebrated anaesthetist, Llewellyn Powell, is demonstrating the use of the Vernon–Harcourt chloroform inhaler.
Reproduced by kind permission of the Queen Square Library, Archive, and Museum, London.

predicted the site of the seizure focus, by correlating the patient's symptoms with his findings on functional anatomy in the monkey, and when he operated found a tuberculoma (a mass of tissue infected by tuberculosis) in the expected position. He completely removed the lesion and also used an induction current to carry out what was in fact the first case of peroperative electrical cortical mapping. In August 1886, Horsley presented the results of his three first cases to a meeting of the British Medical Association in Brighton. Charcot was present and commented that 'British surgery was to be highly congratulated on the recent advances made in the surgery of the nervous system. … Not only had English surgeons cut out tumours of the brain, but here was a case in which it was probable that epilepsy had been cured by operative measures'. By

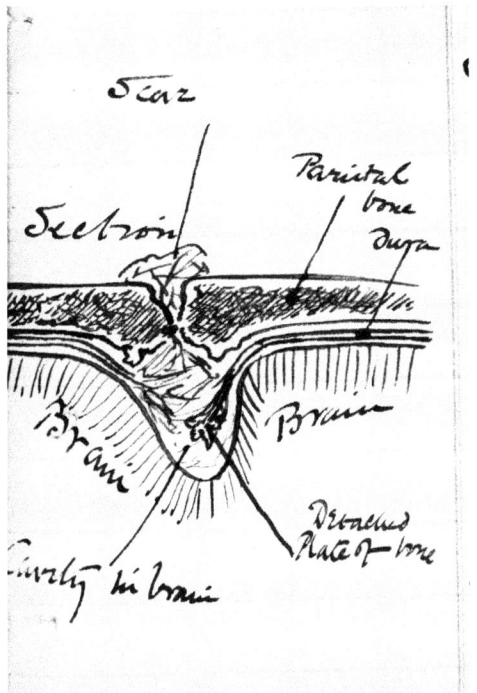

Figure 5.2 A sketch by Horsley of the findings at his first epilepsy operation. Reproduced by kind permission of the Queen Square Library, Archive, and Museum, London.

the end of 1886, Horsley had completed ten epilepsy operations and nine were deemed successful. This was the beginning of epilepsy surgery.

Not only did Horsley carry out quite remarkable experimental work and advance the theories of epilepsy surgery, but he was a brilliant technical surgeon and innovator. He invented methods of opening the skull, methods of stemming blood loss (with bone wax), created new surgical instruments, pioneered the development of a stereotactic frame[6] (the Horsley–Clarke stereotaxic frame), and published stereotaxic atlases of the brain that were far ahead of his time. He continued to operate throughout his life and when his own son Siward suddenly developed convulsions in his late teens, as he was the only surgeon with sufficient skill and experience, he decided to carry out the operation himself. Siward survived the operation, but the seizures recurred.

Neurosurgery was a very small field in those days and dominated by a few pioneering figures. The greatest surgeon of the post-Horsley generation was perhaps Harvey Cushing. He popularised a particular approach to neurosurgery, and also trained many surgeons in his methods, but was not particularly interested in epilepsy. In Germany, two surgeons, Fedor Krause (1857–1937) and then Otfrid Foerster (1871–1943), both pursued epilepsy surgery using electrical stimulation and cortical resections as Horsley had done, but when Horsley was killed in active service in the First World War, epilepsy surgery rather entered the doldrums. The number of epilepsy operations carried out worldwide in the inter-war period was small and the results of surgery failed to live up to its early promise. In the 1920s, Foerster was perhaps the most active epilepsy surgeon of the period, but had become a lonely voice in the tangled jungle of neurosurgery.

The principles underlying this early surgery were that: (i) epilepsy arises from a focal area in the cerebral cortex (that can be predicted by the nature of the seizure symptomatology) and (ii) resecting this area will 'cure' the epilepsy. These two principles have underpinned all subsequent resective surgery of epilepsy to this day, and it is a rather sobering fact there has been no paradigmatic changes since the 1880s in this regard. However, whether either principle is grounded in scientific reality is highly questionable, as is discussed further below.

The next major step in the development of epilepsy surgery had to wait until after the introduction of electroencephalography (EEG) in the late 1930s and with this new technology, the anatomical focus of surgical attention switched from the central neocortex to the temporal lobe. It was Hughlings Jackson who first described the temporal lobe seizure. He named the symptoms the 'dreamy state' and inferred that these arose in the region of the uncinate gyrus (part of the temporal lobe of the brain). His most detailed description was of a patient, Dr 'Z', a medical doctor who had intractable temporal lobe epilepsy and who died from suicide 10 years later. Jackson urged the pathologist carrying out the autopsy 'to search the taste region of Ferrier on each half of the brain very carefully' and as Jackson had predicted, a lesion was found in the uncinate gyrus.[7] In the years prior to EEG, this form of epilepsy was thought to be an unusual curiosity and was a topic which attracted little attention. The introduction of EEG changed this totally, and temporal lobe epilepsy is today considered one of the commonest forms of epilepsy and one which features prominently in contemporary surgical practice (Figure 5.3).

EEG is a remarkable invention which itself has an interesting history. In 1875, Richard Caton[8] showed that there was electrical activity in the brain. In 1890, Adolf Beck, a Polish physiologist showed this oscillated, and introduced the term 'brain waves'. In 1912, Russian physiologists published photographs of animal EEGs, but it was in 1924 that the German physiologist Hans Berger[9] (1873–1941) recorded the first human EEG. Berger showed that it was possible to visualise the brain's electrical activity (human brain waves) on a device

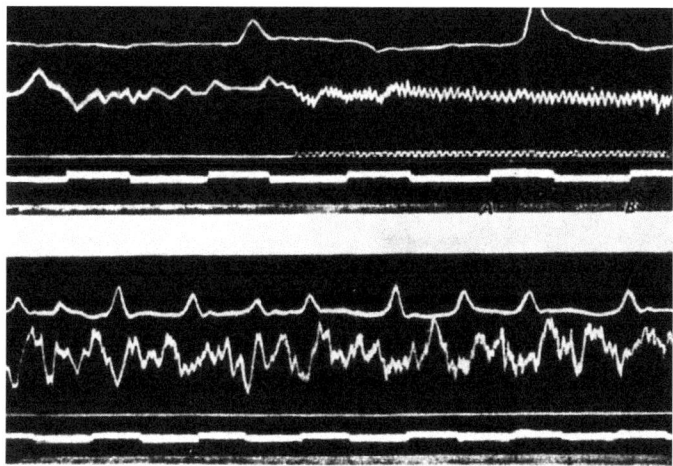

Figure 5.3 The first published EEG trace.
Reproduced with permission from Brazier MAB. (1959/1960) The EEG in Epilepsy—A Historical Note. *Epilepsia*, Volume 1, Issue 1–5, pp. 328–336, Copyright © 1959 John Wiley and Sons.

he called the electroencephalogram, a discovery that was largely ignored until E. D. Adrian[10] and B. H. C. Matthews confirmed Berger's findings and extended his work, in a famous paper in 1934. In 1935, Gibbs, Davis, Jasper, and Lennox started their own work correlating EEG and clinical signs in epilepsy. They described EEG changes both during seizures and interictally. In 1936, the first clinical EEG laboratory opened at Massachusetts General Hospital in Boston. Attention then turned to the potential utility of EEG in epilepsy surgery. Prior to EEG, the only investigations that could be carried out to localise a lesion in epilepsy were air ventriculography and air encephalography, introduced by Walter Dandy in 1918 and 1919, and cerebral angiography introduced in 1926 by Egaz Moniz.[11] These had limited sensitivity and did not show up the small lesions or atrophies in the temporal lobe which most commonly caused epilepsy. In 1941, Jasper and Kershman described the interictal EEG correlates of the temporal lobe seizure and in 1947, Gibbs and colleagues reiterated that the temporal lobe seizure was associated with a specific EEG pattern, 'a focus of spikes at the tip of the temporal lobe'. It was then only a matter of time before a surgeon would be tempted to resect a temporal lobe, and so it was. The first such resections, based entirely on clinical seizure descriptions and EEG recordings showing temporal spikes, were probably carried out by the surgeon Percival Bailey (1892–1973) who reported, with Gibbs, a series of cases in 1951. In 1950,[12] from Montreal, Wilder Penfield (Figure 5.4) had also reported, with Flanigin, a series of 68 cases, it is said based mainly on structural

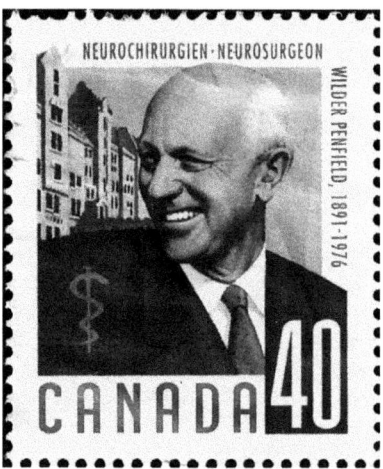

Figure 5.4 Wilder Penfield depicted on a Canadian stamp.
© Her Majesty the Queen in Right of Canada, as represented by Canada Post, 1991.

changes identified by angiography and air encephalography, and in the same year Arthur Morris had presented a series of five temporal lobe resections at a conference in Washington. Although Bailey was the first to resect the temporal lobe cortex, Morris was probably the first to remove the hippocampus as well as the anterior temporal lobe.[13] Both Bailey and Penfield had initially carried out only neocortical resection, and claimed good results, although subsequent experience shows that cortical resection alone in the temporal lobe is not often effective; clearly Bailey and Penfield were erring on the side of 'optimism', and had more objective outcomes actually been reported, it is quite possible that temporal lobectomy would not have generated much interest. As it was, the reports attracted worldwide attention, and temporal lobectomy was taken up in other centres in Europe and North America. By 1952, Penfield had re-operated on his surgical failures and removed the hippocampal structures.

Wilder Penfield was the most celebrated epilepsy surgeon of the period. He had obtained his medical degree at Johns Hopkins, won a Rhodes scholarship to study neurophysiology with Sherrington in Oxford, and did his surgical studies under Cushing in Boston, and during his time in Europe visited Breslau where he was introduced to cortical stimulation by Foerster. When he took up the Directorship of the new Montreal Neurologic Institute in 1934, he pursued his interest in epilepsy. He published, with Herbert Jasper, the landmark book *Epilepsy and the Functional Anatomy of the Human Brain* in 1951, and in this introduced the concept of the 'homunculus' which although it caught the public imagination, in fact added only a small amount of extra knowledge to the cortical maps that Horsley had created decades earlier. He started a programme of temporal lobe epilepsy surgery characterised by careful cortical stimulation, and the extensive use of preoperative and peroperative EEG provided by Jasper. He pioneered 'awake craniotomy' in which, after the brain had been exposed in the first part of an operation, the anaesthesia would be reversed and the patient awakened. He then stimulated the temporal lobe electrically and asked the patient to explain what he or she was experiencing. He sought in this way to mimic the 'aura' of the patient's habitual seizure and to find out from which part of the temporal lobe this arose from. Having thus localised 'the source of the fit', Penfield would resect the cortical tissue in the hope of ameliorating the epilepsy. The underlying theory of resection of the epileptic focus was exactly the same that Horsley adopted in the motor areas of the cerebral cortex. Penfield was also intrigued to find that temporal lobe stimulation produced 'memories' and he thought he had located the seat of memory in the brain, and also mapped accurately the cortical areas relating to speech. It was Penfield who put epilepsy surgery into the forefront of neurosurgery, and the temporal lobectomy has since remained the commonest performed and in many ways the most successful of all surgical procedures for epilepsy.

In London, Murray Falconer, a New Zealander trained by Cairns in the Cushing tradition, was appointed in 1950 as neurosurgeon at the Maudsley Hospital,[14] and had started a surgical programme in which the 'en bloc temporal lobe' resection was designed and performed. This allowed complete pathological examination of the hippocampus and made clear the importance of hippocampal sclerosis (scarring of the mesial temporal lobe) as an underlying pathology, the 'fatal flaw' as it was later termed by the psychiatrist in the team, David Taylor. Falconer and his colleagues provided very detailed reports of diagnosis, psychiatric issues, and surgery, and with the extensive series of Penfield in Montreal, together they established the temporal lobectomy as the major therapeutic advance of its period. As Falconer wrote optimistically in 1954 (13): 'We are now on the threshold of a wide expansion in our knowledge, understanding, and therapeutic control of this ancient scourge of mankind …'.

EEG continued to advance, with various refinement of technique over the next 20 years, which can be only briefly mentioned here. With surgery for epilepsy came the development of EEG recordings within the brain tissue itself or on the surface of the brain and not simply the scalp. Bickford and Cairns in Oxford had performed the first direct incracranial recordings in 1944 in head-injured solders, and Talairach and Bancaud in Paris began inserting depth EEG electrodes using stereotactic procedures in the late 1950s. Crandall and colleagues in California in 1963 then reported the first use of long-term EEG recorded deep in the brain by implanted electrodes, and also established the first EEG video-telemetry unit in 1971. All these developments were important in laying the foundations for our current practice and subsequent physiological advances, but have been incremental rather than paradigmatic. A significant contribution of Talairach and Bancaud in Paris was the evolution of stereotactic methods for localising EEG discharges using depth electrodes based on their celebrated stereotactic atlas of the brain (14). This technique provides a robust method for recording stereo-EEG (SEEG), and has spawned a Franco-Italian school of epilepsy surgery which to this day places enormous emphasis on a detailed analysis of seizure symptoms and EEG and linking this to anatomical data. The theory behind the stereotactic approach was in essence similar to that of Horsley and later Penfield, but Talairach and his colleagues added detailed electrophysiological data. They developed the idea of the epileptogenic zone in 1965 (15) although it should be noted that this term had actually been used by Jackson 100 years earlier, and this concept is discussed further below.

The hemispherectory was another operation applied to epilepsy. This was first carried out by Dandy in 1923 for the resection of a glioma, and used to treat epilepsy in South Africa by Rowland Anthony Krynauw[15] in 1951 who reported its value in 12 children with infantile hemiplegia and epilepsy. The early operations consisted of resecting most of the grey matter of one hemisphere, and were known as anatomical hemispherectomy. The resection left a large potential 'empty' cavity, and unfortunately years later it became clear that this operation was complicated by slow leakage of blood into this space causing what was known as haemosiderosis and hydrocephalus, disastrous complications resulting in severe, progressive, and untreatable disability and eventually death. As a result the operation was largely abandoned. Variants of the anatomical operation were then devised, including the Adams' operation in which the potential space was created outside the coverings of the brain (extradurally). In the 1990s, 'functional' hemispherotomy was introduced with variants proposed by Delalande in 1992, Comair in 1992, and Villemure in 1995. The functional operations do not remove large amounts of tissue but undercut the cortex, thereby removing its connections from the rest of the brain and body. Leaving the isolated brain tissue *in situ* avoids creating a cavity and prevents the occurrence of the late complications. However, the leaving *in situ* of large areas of viable, potentially sentient and conscious but disconnected cortex, must have ethical implications. The variants of the anatomical and functional hemispherectomies all aim to remove (or disconnect) large swathes of cortex in one cerebral hemisphere and as such are the largest brain resections possible to carry out. The operations are obviously applicable only where there is little normal functioning brain tissue in the hemisphere to be resected. Although often effective in controlling epilepsy, the children (for it is usually children in whom the surgery is carried out) are left with multiple neurological problems. It can be a life-saving operation in certain severe infantile epilepsies and still has a place in treatment, but is mutilating and the control of seizures is achieved only at a price.

Splitting the corpus callosum, which is the main fibre tract in the brain carrying messages from one cerebral hemisphere to the other, is not a 'resective' operation but a 'disconnective' one. The idea is to separate (disconnect) the epileptic area in one hemisphere and thus limit the spread of discharges from that hemisphere to the other. The corpus callosectomy was first carried out by Dandy for a cortical cyst, and for epilepsy by van Wagenen and Herren in 1940. Other reports followed, and particularly influential were those of Bogen and colleagues in the 1960s. The operation could be carried in two stages: by the severance of only the anterior fibres initially, followed by a second operation to complete the callosotomy if the initial operation was ineffective, or by a complete callosotomy ab initio. It creates 'a split brain' where in certain circumstances one hemisphere has no information about activity in the other hemisphere, thus creating a wonderful opportunity for weird psychological experiments producing a profusion of esoteric psychological findings. Furthermore, as has been the case with all disconnective operations, the realisation has slowly dawned that the initial reports of good epilepsy control following the procedures were over-optimistic, and in fact, especially in the longer term, most of these operations have proved futile. Enthusiasts still maintain that the benefits of the operation outweigh the drawbacks, but it is now an operation that is only very seldom performed.

Another disconnective operation that enjoyed a brief vogue was multiple subpial transection (sometimes called the Morrell procedure after its originator). This involved the formation of parallel rows of cortical incisions 4–5 mm deep, over the area of the epileptic focus, producing an effect on the brain surface similar to that of a ploughed field. The theoretical basis is that the transections sever the horizontal connections between brain cells and thus prevent the recruitment of neighbouring neurons essential for the production of synchronised epileptic discharges, and yet at the same time preserve normal functions as these are largely served by vertically oriented fibres. This is the theory, but in practice it is not clear whether improvements in epilepsy are due simply to non-specific damage to the cortex caused by the procedure itself. The underpinning theory allows the operation to be carried out in brain areas where resection would result in significant neurological deficit, and it has thus been principally applied to patients with epileptic foci in the primary motor, sensory, and language areas of the brain. Again, early enthusiasm for this approach has not been maintained, and it seems both that seizure control is less good and functional damage is greater than hoped. It is now seldom performed alone, although is still used in combination with a lesion resection in areas in or adjacent to eloquent cortex.

Developments in anaesthesia and in pre- and postoperative care have rendered epilepsy surgery much safer than it was in earlier periods, and in terms of operative technique one significant advance was the introduction of the operating microscope in 1957. In the field of epilepsy surgery, this led to more precise and safer surgery and also allowed surgeons to experiment with different operative approaches, for example, the new approach to hippocampectomy of Yaşargil. Another procedure, radiosurgery (i.e. the application of radiation to destroy tissue in place of surgical resection) using stereotactic methods was introduced by Leksell in 1951 evolving into the so-called gamma knife by Leksell in 1968, which although beloved of newspapers and tickling the public imagination (as 'laser surgery'), has not in epilepsy practice proved superior to the surgeon's knife.

The next paradigm shift in the field of investigation of patients for epilepsy surgery was the introduction of computed X-ray tomography (CT) by Hounsfield in 1967 and then magnetic resonance imaging (MRI) by Mansfield in 1977,[16] technologies which revolutionised many fields of medicine and both of which rightly resulted in a clutch of Nobel Prizes. These 'neuroimaging' techniques provide direct visualisation of brain tissue for the first time, and MRI particularly has such fine resolution, that as the technique has been refined, it can detect lesions and anomalies of brain structures of less than 1 cm in size. The consequences for epilepsy surgery have been profound. MRI provides more certainty and more accuracy for detecting and localising lesions and has been a great boost for this, as all other, neurosurgical procedures. The sensitivity and specificity of MRI have been progressively improved by new software and hardware developments including the use of higher and higher magnetic field strengths, new imaging sequences tailored to the types of pathologies seen in epilepsy, volumetric imaging where 3D 'volume' data is collected, post-processing, co-registration of the localisation data from EEG and MRI and other imaging modalities in 3D space, magnetic resonance angiography, and functional imaging of blood flow. Each has contributed to improvements in practice, and a detailed consideration of this is outside the scope of this book. The excitement of MRI also resulted in renewed interest in the underlying structural changes in epilepsy, and to some extent a switch of emphasis to structure (MRI) from function (EEG). MRI also allowed the identification of lesions which previously were invisible and unexpected as causes of epilepsy such as cavernoma or cortical dysplasia, and provides visual and quantitative evidence of hippocampal sclerosis. In the wake of MRI, the concept of 'lesionectomy' has arisen, that is, a resection of the lesion only and not surrounding tissue, as a way of minimising adverse effects. MRI provides exquisite pictures of a lesion and its anatomical position, and opens the possibility not only of a conventional surgical resection under direct vision, but also too of stereotactic lesionectomy, controlled by automated computerised computation of the position of the lesion in stereotactic space.

Other new technologies have found a place in investigation including functional MRI (fMRI), single-photon emission computed tomography (SPECT), and positron emission tomography (PET) scanning.[17] These each create attractive colour pictures with which to formulate a case or adorn a publication, but it is not clear to us in what proportion of patients these technologies actually change treatment or improve outcome. These are areas, along with invasive EEG, in which specificity and sensitivity studies need to be performed, and health utilisation or health technology evaluation carried out.

Finally, 'brain stimulation' should be mentioned. This is a totally different surgical strategy used in epilepsy since the 1930s. The idea is that by delivering trains of electrical stimulation to certain areas of the brain, the synchrony or development of an epileptic seizure can somehow be prevented. In intracranial stimulation, brain areas are stimulated directly via intracranial electrodes placed into the brain substance. In the 1930s, the areas targeted included the amygdala, various thalamic nuclei, the fields of Forel, the anterior commissure, the fornix, and the posterior limb of the internal capsule. The results of these operations were generally poor and this type of functional surgery lingered but then largely faded out by the 1950s. In the last decade, though, interest has been rekindled in the technique rebranded as 'deep brain stimulation' (DBS). This initiative has been justified by the much improved anatomical precision of MRI-guided stereotaxy, better stimulation technology, safer implantation, and also by the success of these procedures in other conditions such as Parkinson's disease and in pain. The targets which have been studied include the caudate nucleus, the centromedian nucleus of the thalamus, the anterior thalamic nucleus, the mammillary bodies, and the subthalamic nucleus, and also direct stimulation of the epileptic focus, in both the neocortex and the hippocampus. The frequency, pattern, and intensity of the electrical stimulation can be varied. More recently, stimulators have been devised that are switched on only when epileptic seizures, recorded by implanted electrodes, start to develop. Whether many of these techniques will be of enduring value is not yet clear. The same might apply to what surely is the strangest of all the stimulation vogues, of stimulation of nerves outside the brain with the intention of sending trains of impulses backwards up the nerves to the brain and thereby in some mysterious way inhibiting the epileptic seizure. Stimulation of the vagus nerve in the neck is the most common example, and trials purport to show an effect. Of course, this does not involve a neurosurgical operation, and so the procedure is inherently attractive to patients and doctors who are suspicious of the risks of direct brain stimulation. Due largely to extensive marketing, the use of vagal nerve stimulation has grown rapidly and in the first 10 years after its introduction in 1997, around 50 000 patients had been treated. Most, but not all, studies have been uncontrolled and some studies have shown an observable, albeit modest, effect. Since then, stimulation of the trigeminal nerve and other nerves has also been claimed to have an effect. The authors' personal and anecdotal experience in all these techniques though has been disappointing.

The Theoretic Basis of Epilepsy Surgery

Underpinning all modern resective surgery has been the process of 'presurgical assessment'. At the heart of this assessment is the bringing together of the results from neuroimaging, neurophysiological, and neuropsychological investigations and their integration with the seizure symptomatology and other neurological and psychiatric findings. The idea has grown up that the more 'congruent' are the findings of this assessment, the more likely is the outcome of surgery to be good. Congruent cases are those in which all modalities of the assessment point to dysfunction in the same area of the brain. Unfortunately, there is an increasing tendency to add test after test to the mix, including functional imaging and depth EEG and the idea of congruence becomes increasingly less easy to evaluate. The virtues of the principle of 'lining the ducks all in a row' is often enunciated, but this is intellectually banal.

As emphasised throughout this chapter, the concept of resective surgery depends on two particular principles: (i) epileptic seizures have a focal origin, which can be identified on the basis of the clinical features and the results of EEG and imaging investigations; and (ii) resection of the focus will result in the 'cure' of the epilepsy. It is worth further considering these points.

The idea that the epileptic seizure starts in a small focal area of the brain is problematic, and might be termed the *phrenological fallacy*. The naïve imagery, often portrayed of the origin of a seizure and its spread, is of the point where a stone is thrown into the water of a pond (the origin) and of the ripples extending out through the pond (the spread). However, it is abundantly clear from many different lines of evidence, that this simplistic view of the physiology of a 'seizure' is patently incorrect, at least for the majority of seizures. Many do not start in a small focal area but are the result of activation of a whole network of cells (in the latest jargon—a neural network) with activation sometimes simultaneously seen in different parts of the network or in varying alternative parts of the network in different seizures.[18] The fact that the clinical features of a temporal lobe seizure involve many aspects which are not part of temporal lobe function (motor aspects, loss of consciousness, etc.) and the very commonly observed fact of the persistence of auras after temporal lobe surgery, even if full-blown complex partial seizures are controlled, are demonstrations of how, whatever is achieved by resective surgery, it cannot be the removal of the focal onset.

Along with the concept of congruence have arisen the concepts of the 'epileptogenic zone', the 'symptomatic zone', the 'irritative zone', and the 'ictal onset zone'. Spencer (18) provides a definition of an epileptogenic network as: 'a functionally and anatomically connected, bilaterally represented, set of cortical and subcortical brain structures and regions in which activity in any one part affects activity in all the others' and that 'vulnerability to seizure activity in any one part of the network is influenced by activity everywhere else in the network ... the network as a whole is responsible for the clinical and electrographic phenomena that we associate with human seizures'. This is indubitably the case, and in passing it is interesting to note that what is true of an epileptic seizure is probably also true of many higher brain functions, which explains why efforts to localise higher functions in the brain (as opposed to the primary motor and sensory functions) have been doomed to failure. The continuing tendency to view the brain as the phrenologists did (with a love centre, a memory centre, a music centre, etc.) has proved pointless and naïve.

In limbic epilepsy (temporal lobe epilepsy), structural, functional, and metabolic studies all demonstrate widespread alterations in networks in both limbic and non-limbic areas. Experimentally, the onset of a focal seizure is characterised by a whole variety of different changes, some widespread. These include disinhibitory and hypersynchronous activity, oscillatory changes, and state changes which can be seen relatively focally and also in more widespread, even non-adjacent areas and sometimes in similar areas in both hemispheres. Much of this phenomenology is poorly understood, but its widely distributed nature is clear and this particularly applies to temporal lobe seizures (better termed limbic seizures to emphasise the network aspects). Lesional epilepsy in the neocortex, especially the central neocortex, may have a more focal onset and the epilepsy focus maybe quite localised as shown for instance in the small area of type IIb cortical dysplasia, from which the epileptic activity arises, or from a small cavernoma or tumour.

If this is the case, it could be asked why surgery which removes only part of the network ever stops seizures? One answer may be that it damages or degrades a network sufficiently to inhibit the processes leading to the clinical seizure. This would explain the maxim, well known to epilepsy surgeons, that the bigger the resection, the more likely is epilepsy to cease ('more is better', as the celebrated epilepsy surgeon from Montreal, Rasmussen, used to say). Another interesting, and disappointing phenomenon, is that the initial seizure-suppressive effects of any surgery has a tendency to wear off, and the epilepsy recurs over time in increasing number of cases. The most parsimonious explanation of this curious fact is that the underpinning network, which was degraded or disconnected by surgery, is reorganised by processes of cerebral plasticity, and these (maladaptive) processes restore epileptogenicity. If this is the case, then a better understanding might lead in the future to post-surgical therapies aimed at inhibiting these developments. The fact that antiepileptic drug treatment does often need to be continued, even if seizures have ceased after surgery, is another phenomenon which suggests that surgery does not remove a focus, but simply weakens or degrades the tendency for seizures to develop.

The *phrenological fallacy* explains why 'presurgical assessment' carried out to 'find the focus' is a procedure based on faulty premises in many cases. While it is obviously important to localise the extent of the network or 'epileptogenic zone' as much as possible, it is wrong to consider that the surgical outcome depends on the removal of a focus in most cases. For some seizures, especially those associated with neocortical vascular or tumoural lesions or small focal dysplasias, it is probably the case that there are limited foci of epileptogenicity, but this is not the case for most temporal lobe epilepsies or for the epilepsies associated with no observable cortical lesion (the 'MRI-negative' cases). Thus, the current tendency to add investigation after investigation to the assessment of a patient seems to us to be misplaced, in a search for an illusory "focus" in what is essentially a network phenomenon. Technically intriguing such investigations may be, producing elegant and often visually attractive results, there seems little real comparative evidence that they improve the outcome of surgery.

Outcome of Epilepsy Surgery

The preceding sections of this chapter have been concerned with the historical development of epilepsy surgery and its theoretical basis, and now we turn to outcome. There is no doubt, as Horsley himself hoped, that outstanding results can be obtained, and that the lives of many patients, whose epilepsy was previously impervious to drug therapy, can be immeasurably improved by appropriate surgical treatment. However, for various reasons, the potential benefits have received more of the oxygen of publicity than the potential risks, and in this final section, a deliberately more sceptical and critical appraisal is taken. Perhaps we over-emphasise the downside, but we do so in the spirit of Janus, looking forward as well as back.

The outcome of epilepsy surgery of course depends on the type of operation and the indications for surgery. Sometimes the operation is needed partly to deal with the underlying pathology itself, in addition to the epilepsy (for instance, in the case of cerebral tumour), and sometimes the surgery is carried out in the recognition that this is not likely to control seizures but might ameliorate them, for instance, with brain stimulation or disconnective operations. Usually, however, the desired outcome is seizure freedom and the risks of surgery need to be balanced against the chance of the operation succeeding.

The results of surgery depend a great deal on the anatomical area being operated upon. The most commonly undertaken, and indeed probably the most successful of the curative surgical procedures for epilepsy, is the temporal lobectomy. Although different variants have been devised, the results of these are in general terms no different from that of the standard operation. Whichever variant is chosen, it is important not to give the impression that the operation guarantees long-term seizure control. Most operations have an excellent result but certainly not all, and there has been a marked tendency amongst neurosurgeons, and also the surgery aficionados among neurologists, to make unsubstantiated claims which are not in fact supported by the literature. In fact, at 1 year post-surgery, in published studies, 'seizure freedom' rates have generally ranged between 50% and 80% (median 70%), but at 10 years, rates have ranged between 30% and 60%. The most comprehensive study of nearly 500 patients following temporal lobectomies shows at 5 years that about 50% of patients remained free of seizures with loss of consciousness and the figure falls to about one-third at 10 years after the operation. Furthermore, 'seizure free' in this, as in many, series includes patient who continue to have auras or simple partial seizures. Of course, many patients improve even if they are not rendered seizure free, although about 20% of patients continue to have at least one seizure a month. The results of temporal lobe surgery also depend on the underlying aetiology, and are better for complete hippocampal resection than partial resection (more is better again) and also if the patient has a history of only complex partial seizures and no convulsive seizures prior to surgery (convulsive seizures can be taken as indicating a more extensive network). Epilepsy surgery outside the temporal lobe has a significantly worse outlook, and with rates of medium-term seizure control commonly around 20–30%, but there are very few long-term studies.

It is a striking fact that, in contrast to drug therapy, there is no regulatory approval process for assessing whether surgical treatment is better than non-surgical treatment or no treatment. Invariably today, a surgical procedure is developed in one centre, the results are published as a clinical observation and other surgeons try it without control. There is in fact, a single randomised controlled study of temporal lobectomy showing that this has a better short-term outcome than drug therapy alone, but there are no controlled studies of other forms of resective surgery. There has also been one study using 'sham controls' which was carried out in traumatic epilepsy, by Penfield and Jasper in 1954. In a series of 76 patients with traumatic epilepsy, 59 were routinely operated on with cortical excision and in 16 sham surgery was performed by doing a craniotomy only (opening the skull without touching the brain). The sham surgery resulted in a seizure reduction of 50% in 5 of the 16 cases (32%) but none became seizure free (19). The randomised controlled study referred to above showed that the overall results of temporal lobectomy are better, in terms of seizure control, than those of not operating and continuing treatment only with drugs; however, this benefit has to be balanced against the potential side effects of surgery. This is not always an easy balance to weigh, not least as much is not known about some types of behavioural side effects nor of the long-term adverse effects of operation. Furthermore, while most drug-induced side effects reverse when the drug is withdrawn, the effects of surgery are permanent.

Side effects of epilepsy surgery are of various types. There are immediate risks of stroke and even death, but these are small and the rate of major catastrophes should not exceed 1% in any modern unit. There is also a risk to visual fields of about 5% but this is not often of major import. More serious and well studied are the effects on memory and the risk of postoperative psychiatric disturbance. The temporal lobes are thought to be involved in memory, mood, and behaviour and so such adverse effects would not be unexpected; indeed, perhaps more surprising is the fact that these are not more frequent or more severe. Postoperative memory defects are common but usually mild or moderate and a profound amnesia occurs in less than 1% of cases in modern practice. Memory has been focused upon ever since the case of 'HM', operated upon in 1953 and left with a profound anterograde amnesia.[19] The risks to memory have been well studied, and the degree to which memory loss will occur can be now predicted with reasonable accuracy. However, what is not clear is to what extent temporal lobectomy renders the person more vulnerable to further deterioration in memory functions later in life due to loss of what is known as 'cerebral reserve'. Suggestions that this is the case have been made, but no robust data exist and this is an area deserving of more study.

A greater and less predictable risk after temporal lobectomy is postoperative psychiatric disturbance. In early series, the incidence of schizophreniform illness following temporal lobectomy was about 15%, but in recent studies the incidence of *de novo* psychosis following temporal lobe surgery is much lower, less than 5%, mainly because surgery is now not carried out in patients with a history of psychosis. A depressive illness following temporal lobectomy is more common, occurring in about 35% of patients in the first year after surgery and the incidence of all psychiatric disease is higher in those who are not seizure free following surgery; and patients with postoperative seizures and psychotic illness pose grave problems for postoperative rehabilitation.

Other adverse effects on behaviour and personality have hardly been explored in any systematic fashion. This is true of temporal lobectomy as well as other types of resective and disconnective surgeries, and is a grievous omission. Furthermore, the history of neurosurgery has an unfortunate precedent in this regard, that of the frontal lobotomy, which was an operation introduced in the 1930s for the treatment of severe psychiatric disorders. It became widely performed (over 70 000 operations were carried out) and Egas Moniz, its originator, won the Nobel Prize for Medicine for his work.[20] It was claimed to be effective in 50–80% of patients operated, and many patients 'praised' the operation in the lay press. However, severe cognitive and behavioural side effects were then identified which had not been initially noticed largely because no one had looked. Some patients became docile, devoid of initiative or of emotionality, and sank into a state of isolation and torpor. The operation is now widely condemned, both professionally and also in the public mind,[21] for a flawed physiological basis, for its destructive effects on brain function, and in particular for the lack of care in defining or understanding its adverse effects. It is now hardly ever carried out. Although the operation was sometimes dramatically succesfull, the cure rates claimed were optimistic and the side effects were underplayed; there are obvious lessons here for epilepsy surgery, and it is important that in our quest to find cures for devastating epilepsy that we do not fall into the same trap.

A unilateral temporal lobectomy will remove approximately 10% of the total cerebral cortical volume. Large frontal lobectomy may remove up to 20% of functioning cortex, and both will disconnect important and widespread tracts. It is inconceivable that such large resections have no effect on higher brain function. Although the incidence of depression and psychosis and the frequency and severity of memory deficits after temporal lobectomy are well studied, almost no other cognitive or behavioural effects have been systematically studied. It is vital that this is rectified, not least as patients have a right to be fully counselled on these effects. The omission is difficult to understand or justify, not least because there is abundant animal experimentation demonstrating effects on various aspects of behaviour.

The classic primate experiments of Kluver and Bucy, for instance, demonstrated a range of remarkable effects on sexuality and aggression after temporal lobe resection, without any alteration of intelligence, memory, or motor function. In the early days of the Maudsley series, Pond and his colleagues carried out a study of sexuality after temporal lobectomy. Many patients were at this time selected because of high degrees of psychiatric disturbance, but their findings were nevertheless interesting. They reported that after temporal lobectomy, a change in the intensity of libido or in its direction and choice of object was noted in 14/16 patients (88%). In the only other systematic study, Baird and colleagues in Melbourne surveyed sexual function in 58 patients after temporal lobectomy and 16 after extratemporal lobe resections and concluded that the majority of the temporal lobe cases reported a postoperative sexual change; 45% of patients reported an increase in sexual drive, often with thoughts and fantasies 'many times a day'. Florid cases exhibited massive increases in masturbatory behaviour. A smaller number described hyposexual changes, and of course, this is similar to what Kluver and Bucy observed in their experiments in rhesus monkeys. Obsessionality is another trait that has been reported to be altered in isolated case reports after epilepsy surgery. Several extreme case reports have been published of repetitive sexual, religious, and obscene thoughts, extreme cleaning and repeating behaviours, excessive hand washing, an obsessive and compulsive security checking, concern about filth and germs, a fear of being hurt, compulsive reorganising behaviour, and repetitive touching. Another behaviour which has been known for many years to be affected after temporal lobe resection is aggressiveness, but again this has received no systematic study in the epilepsy field. Golz noted in 1890 that removing the temporal lobe in a dog reduced aggression, and Kluver and Bucy noted a marked reduction in aggressiveness in their monkeys. In humans, bilateral amygdalohippocampectomies (removal of the amygdala and hippocampus) were once carried out specifically to reduce aggressiveness. Narabayashi reported a marked improvement in 'emotional excitability' in 60 patients in his series, and Pond noted a similar change in all 12 patients in his series who had had aggressive tendencies before temporal lobe surgery. The fact is that if temporal lobectomy results in 'taming', then the patients should be counselled accordingly, but in our experience this is hardly ever done. Most of the above-described effects have been related to temporal lobe surgery and there is very little information about the effects of extratemporal lobe surgery on any high level cortical function. One trait which has been studied is that of musical appreciation. Various case reports of all types of effect have been reported and we have personally observed patients becoming effectively tone death following neocortical resection.

The above-mentioned features represent only a small sample of aspects of human behaviour, emotion, and cognition which could be studied, and are in some senses illustrative only.

The main points we want to make are that there are many functions, behavioural, sexual, emotional, and cognitive, which are known to be affected by epilepsy surgery, and yet the frequency and extent of impairment is not known.

These are furthermore seldom discussed with the patient and are seldom assessed after surgery, and yet are features which can have a major effect on psychosocial functioning and quality of life. The lack of knowledge on these points is highly regrettable. The lack of counselling on these points is even worse, and is, in the view of some authorities, unethical.

Studies are no doubt difficult as the extent of such effects will be affected by premorbid psychological and psychiatric status, the site and extent of the resection, the preoperative personality, and the level of brain function. Nevertheless, the situation has certain parallels to that which applied to frontal lobotomy, and although hopefully any effects after epilepsy surgery are less severe, we should be warned by the frontal lobotomy experience. In both types of surgery, the lack of surveillance for, or study of, adverse effects means that some effects can pass under the medical radar.

This is of course not to say that epilepsy surgery should not be carried out. On the contrary, in well-selected cases this is a life-saving therapy, but so was frontal lobotomy. The almost total lack of study of some of these complex psychological or cognitive effects of temporal lobectomy, or of any effect of frontal or other neocortical resection, linked to a tendency to give over-optimistic assessments of seizure outcome, is concerning.

The above narrative has been based on a narrow clinical perspective, and of course there are important societal trends which have had a major impact on the course of epilepsy surgery over this period. One obvious example is the impact of financial considerations. With newer technologies, the increasing potential for profit has not escaped the attention of corporations, and the commercial aspects of epilepsy surgery have become an important consideration in some settings, particularly in the United States. There is also no doubt that large profits can be made with expensive presurgical examination alone, even without subsequent surgery, a not uncommon consequence for epilepsies thought to be arising from outside the temporal lobe. Many centres have sprung up where operations are offered. These are sometimes glossy temples of metal and glass, critics suspect, the clinical work is increasingly dependent on marketing hype. The centres provide video promotions, photographs of 5-star accommodation and smiling staff, and the promise of a happier future. Glowing public utterances and colourful websites and brochures increasingly use advertising techniques, and the marketing risks being unbalanced despite the best efforts of the professional organisations and the regulators to avoid this.

There is a growing concern that not only that this obscures the downsides of surgery, but also that surgical treatment has been exaggerated beyond its importance in the field of epilepsy, to the detriment of other less glamorous aspects of epilepsy. If the social disadvantages of the ordinary patient, or the plight of the handicapped, had had the same profile and marketing skills applied, greater action might have resulted which would have advanced the cause of far more patients. Furthermore, part of the commercial interest has been to stimulate artificial demand. It is frequently claimed that 'surgery should not be the treatment of last resort' and that there are large numbers of patients who would benefit from surgery but who are being denied access to this largely by the sloth of their medical advisors. This seems to us an overblown claim, for while there certainly are patients for whom surgery should be considered, estimates of numbers are often exaggerated. Where surgery is freely offered without the marketing back-up, and where financial pressures are less, the numbers of operated cases has not risen greatly, and indeed it is commonly said that the 'easy' cases (for instance, those with unilateral hippocampal sclerosis and congruent investigatory findings) now are rarely seen. In the United Kingdom, where treatment is free, but which has a relatively conservative approach to surgery, a survey of all neurological units found in 2003 (20) 324 temporal lobe resections, 70 extratemporal lobe resections, 14 hemispherectomies, and 14 corpus callosotomies were performed; a total of 422 neurosurgical procedures and in addition 156 vagal nerve stimulators were inserted. This was considered only a modest increase on the 150 resective operations recorded in 1991. Efforts were then made to increase the number of operated cases, and although accurate comparative figures are not available, it seems likely that there has been little increase. Furthermore, many cases referred for surgery prove unsuitable, for one reason or another, and it seems likely that the pool of unoperated patients in the community contains fewer suitable candidates for surgery than previously claimed.

Wading Through the Hype

So what can be concluded about epilepsy surgery in the modern era? It opened the era with great promise and has become an established therapy. Technology has greatly improved as have the technical aspects of surgery and perioperative care, and these have made the operative procedures much safer. Investigatory technologies have also made a profound difference to epilepsy surgery, first with the advent of EEG and its various developments, and then with the introduction of CT and MRI, the latter particularly providing incredible anatomical detail. Theory though has lagged behind and the theoretical underpinning, at least of resective surgery, remains very similar to that of Horsley and his colleagues who purported to identify the 'epileptogenic zone' using the seizure symptoms, and proposed resection of this tissue as a way of curing epilepsy.

This approach is at the basis of all resective surgery since, and although mounting evidence exists of the diffuse network nature of a seizure, most surgical thought is still entrenched in the idea of removing the focus. If epilepsy surgery, especially of the temporal lobe, acts by interfering with or degrading the epileptic network, rather than resecting a focus, perhaps alternative approaches should be considered. Disconnective surgery such as corpus callosotomy and multiple subpial transection, however, has proved disappointing, and brain stimulation seems largely empirical and as yet has shown only rather limited value. A new paradigm is needed, and it is possible other methods of interfering with epileptic networks will prove beneficial.

An area where technology assessment is urgently needed is in the appropriate choice of investigation carried out as part of the presurgical assessment. The sensitivity and specificity of these remain almost entirely unknown, and it is our impression that there is large redundancy in the tests carried out. To what extent this is simply a lack of rigor or reflects genuine uncertainly is not clear, but evaluation especially of functional imaging and invasive EEG is in our opinion overdue.

The claims about the outcome of almost all types of epilepsy operations, when first carried out, almost always prove too optimistic. It would be preferable for the outcome assessment to be performed by independent agencies and not the surgeons or epilepsy teams whose vested interests are served by the surgery; this leads to unconscious or even conscious bias. In determining the results of drug treatment, regulatory agencies demand stringent checks on data, but this is utterly absent in evaluating surgery. Furthermore, multicentre and transnational data need to be collected, as even the largest surgical centres perform too few cases to make proper statistical judgements. The long-term outcome of many types of surgery remains poorly studied. The effects on surgery on many aspects of cerebral functioning, and the longer-term effects in terms of cerebral reserve, have hardly been looked at, and these are grievous omissions.

Epilepsy surgery is an elective procedure and irreversible, and yet evidence to base risk versus benefit analysis is currently substandard. This is an unsatisfactory situation and something which should be addressed by systematic research. We need to be able to provide detailed objective counselling and currently we are not in a position to do so. While successful epilepsy surgery can be life-changing and life-enhancing, and indeed can produce an almost magical transformation in an afflicted person's predicament, both the prediction of success and the downsides of surgery are uncertain. We should be able to do better than this.

Notes

1. Antisepsis was pioneered by Joseph Lister whose work had a profound effect on surgery worldwide. He was also a key figure in the development of neurosurgery in the sense that McEwan was a colleague of Lister in Glasgow, Rickman Godlee was Lister's nephew, and Horsley was a friend of Lister and was fanatical in his adherence to Listerian methods of antisepsis. Indeed Lister was present at Godlee's and Horsley's earliest operations.
2. Orotracheal intubation is performed by inserting a tube in the throat to protect the passage of air to the lungs during surgery. The idea was not a new one, and, for instance, was described by Versalius, but the modern technique and its use in surgery were first employed by Macewen, see Macmillan (1).
3. James Simpson (1811–1870), William Macewen (1848–1924), and Sir Victor Horsley (1857–1916).
4. Ferrier published his results in two celebrated books (2,3) and dedicated the first work to Jackson.
5. This was a truly remarkable meeting in many ways, and is well described in contemporary diaries and newspapers. See Sakula (4).
6. Stereotactic surgery is a form of operation in which the target for surgery is defined mathematically by a three-dimensional (3D) coordinate system. The stereotactic frame, using a Cartesian (three-orthogonal axis) system, was invented by Clarke and Horsley. The principle and modern design variants of the frame are widely used today in human neurosurgery. The actual frame design Clarke and Horsley invented was still in use in the 1970s—see Schurr and Merrington (5).
7. This case was published (6) and the post-mortem findings published 18 years later (7). In a brilliant piece of medical detective work, the identity of Dr Z was uncovered and he was found to be a Dr Arthur Thomas Myers who died on 10 January 1894, having taken a chloral overdose and who turned out to be a close neighbour and friend of Jackson—see Taylor and Marsh (8).
8. Richard Caton (1842–1926) was a physician in Liverpool.
9. Hans Berger (1873 –1941) was a German psychiatrist and considered the originator of the EEG. Berger though was an outsider, ridiculed and mistrusted by the German scientific and medical establishment, and his findings were largely ignored until confirmed by Adrian and Matthews in 1934. Berger suffered from recurrent depression and committed suicide in 1941.
10. Edgar Douglas Adrian (1889–1977) was a world-renowned Cambridge scientist who was awarded the Nobel Prize in Physiology or Medicine in 1932. It was his confirmation of Berger's findings which led to the interest.
11. Air ventriculography is a performed by injecting air into the ventricles of the brain (fluid-filled spaces in the centre of the mammalian brain). The air is then visualised on X-ray and allows the anatomy of the ventricles to be delineated. Angiography is a method in which a dye is injected into the arteries. The dye is radio-opaque (i.e. causes a 'shadow' on X-ray) and this allows the anatomical position of the arteries of the brain to be delineated. The ventricles or arteries can be pushed out of their normal position by a tumour or other mass, and so these methods allow the surgeon to infer indirectly the position of any abnormal mass in the brain. These tests became obsolete for this purpose when CT and MRI were developed which can directly visualise the mass. Walter Dandy

(1886–1946) was an American neurosurgeon at Johns Hopkins Hospital in Baltimore. Egaz Moniz (1874–1955) was a Portuguese neurologist who won a Nobel Prize, not for the invention of angiography which was an enduring contribution, but for the invention of the operation of frontal lobotomy.

12. The classic papers were by Morris (9) and Penfield and Flanigin (10). The precedence is discussed by Moran (11) and Engel (12).
13. In true surgical style, there has been a battle for precedence about the hippocampal resection along nationalistic line, with the US and Canadian teams both claiming first place. It is probable that hippocampal resection was carried out almost simultaneously by both groups, with Bailey perhaps the originator (11).
14. As was the case in Boston and in Montreal, the importance of having an epilepsy 'team' with different specialities had been this time been recognised as indispensable. At the Maudsley, for instance, Falconer worked with his junior surgeon Peter Schurr, physicians Denis Hill and Desmond Pond, pathologists Alfred Meyer and Nick Corsellis and later C. Bruton, electroencephalographers George Dawson and Maurice Driver, psychiatrist David Taylor, and radiologist R. D. (Dick) Hoare. All were interested in epilepsy.
15. Rowland Anthony Krynauw (1907–1990) trained in medicine in Edinburgh and learned his neurosurgery in Oxford during the Second World War under Cairns and in London, see Anonymous (16).
16. Sir Godfrey Newbold Hounsfield, CBE, FRS (1919–2004), winner of the 1979 Nobel Prize for Physiology or Medicine; Sir Peter Mansfield FRS (b. 1933) winner of the 2003 Nobel Prize in Physiology or Medicine.
17. fMRI is a technique in which the movement of blood is registered on an MRI scan. It works on the theory that when brain regions are activated, more blood flows in the activated area, and so by this technique the MRI scan can pick up areas of activation. The same theory is utilised by SPECT and PET which use CT scanning and radioactive tracers to identify the regions of high blood flow. SPECT particularly is used to identify the 'epileptic focus' during an epileptic seizure (on the basis that during a focal seizure, blood flow is greatly increased in the area of the seizure—the focus).
18. For a review of experimental work in this field, see Jiruska et al. (17).
19. Henry Molaison ('HM') (1926–2008) was a patient with intractable epilepsy, who was treated with a bilateral temporal lobectomy by the Hartford neurosurgeon William Scoville. The operation was carried out when he was aged 27, and following the operation he developed a profound anterograde amnesia such that HM could not form any memories of ongoing events. He was intensively studied by Dr Brenda Milner, a psychologist from Montreal, and his case contributed to much theory about the mechanisms of memory. By virtue of his severe amnesia, he became rather a celebrity, appearing in the media and examined by many curious psychologists.
20. When Moniz was awarded his Nobel Prize, *The New York Times* wrote an enthusiastic editorial about the wonders of frontal lobotomy 'Surgeons now think no more of operating on the brain than they do of removing an appendix. Hess, Moniz and Cushing taught us to look with less awe on the brain. It is just a big organ …. And no more sacred than the liver'. This ridiculous comment reflected the societal attitudes of the time, and general optimism about medicine and technology, no doubt driven in part by financial forces.
21. The operation was vilified in many popular books and films including *One Flew Over the Cuckoo's nest* and *The Bell Jar*.

References

1. **Macmillan M.** William Macewen (1848–1924). *J Neurol* 2010; **257**(5):858–859.
2. **Ferrier D.** *The Functions of the Brain*. London: Smith, Elder & Co; 1876.
3. **Ferrier D.** *Localisation of Cerebral Disease*. London: Smith, Elder & Co; 1878.
4. **Sakula A.** Baroness Burdett-Coutts' garden party: the International Medical Congress, London, 1881. *Med Hist* 1982; **36**:183–190.
5. **Schurr PH, Merrington WR.** The Horsley-Clarke stereotaxic apparatus. *Br J Surg* 1978; **65**:33–36.
6. **Jackson HJ.** On a particular variety of epilepsy ("intellectual aura"), one case with symptoms of organic brain disease. *Brain* 1880; **11**:179–207.
7. **Jackson HJ, Colman WS.** Case of epilepsy with tasting movements and 'dreamy state'-very small patch off softening in the left uncinate gyrus. *Brain* 1898; **21**:580–90.
8. **Taylor DC, Marsh SM.** Hughlings Jackson's Dr Z: the paradigm of temporal lobe epilepsy revealed. *J Neurol Neurosurg Psychiatry* 1980; **43**:758–767.
9. **Morris AA.** The surgical treatment of psychomotor epilepsy. *Med Ann Dist Col* 1950; **119**:121–131.
10. **Penfield W, Flanigin H.** Surgical therapy of temporal lobe seizures. *Arch Neurol Psychiatry* 1950; **64**:491–500.
11. **Moran NF.** A more balanced and inclusive view of the history of temporal lobectomy. *Epilepsia* 2008; **49**:543–544.
12. **Engel JJr.** More on the history of temporal lobe epilepsy. *Epilepsia* 2008; **49**:1481–1482.
13. **Falconer MA.** Clinical manifestations of temporal lobe epilepsy and their recognition in relation to surgical treatment. *Br Med J* 1954; **2**:939–944.
14. **Talairach J, Szikla P, Tournoux A, et al.** *Atlas d'anatomie stéréotaxique du télencéphale: études anatomo-radiologiques*. Paris: Masson; 1967.
15. **Bancaud J, Talairach J, Bonis A, et al.** *La stéréoélectroencéphalographie dans l'épilepsie: informations neurophysiopathologiques apportées par l'investigation fonctionnelle stereotaxique*. Paris: Masson; 1965.
16. **Anonymous.** In memoriam – R.M. Newbery and R.A.H. Krynauw. *S Afr Med J* 1991; **79**(2 Mar):287–288.
17. **Jiruska P, de Curtis M, Jefferys JGR (eds).** Modern concepts of focal epileptic networks. *Int Rev Neurobiol* 2014; **114**: 2–348.
18. **Spencer SS.** Neural networks in human epilepsy: evidence of and implications for treatment. *Epilepsia* 2002; **43**(3):219–227.
19. **Penfield W, Jasper H.** *Epilepsy and the Functional Anatomy of the Human Brain*. Boston, MA: Little, Brown and Company; 1954.
20. **Lhatoo S, Solomon J, McEvoy A, Kitchen N, Shorvon S, Sander J.** A prospective study of the requirement for and the provision of epilepsy surgery in the United Kingdom. *Epilepsia* 2003; **44**(5):673–676.

Chapter 6

The Dark Side of Epilepsy

Epilepsy is a Janus-faced disease. It has a bright and a dark side, and it is the dark side which is the topic of this chapter. For some individuals, seizures are the only health problem, early treatment works, sometimes treatment can be withdrawn after a few years, and a normal life is possible; for these fortunate people, the condition confers only relatively slight and transient inconvenience. However, others are traumatised by the experience of having had seizures, even if these have resolved. For others, however, the condition has a much darker side that can harm and can devastate. In about 20% of individuals, seizures once developed can never be fully controlled by medication (1) and for some, control takes many years or is never achieved (1). When severe, epilepsy can destroy health and shorten life. Treatment can sometimes be denied, delayed, or inappropriately applied, with devastating consequences; mistreatment, over-treatment, or under-treatment all occur. Modern drugs and devices for uncontrolled seizures may offer a poor value proposition. Millions of people are taking drugs that do not help them, have had operations which have failed to stop the seizures, or have had scans or other tests that carry no benefit. Some new drugs have generated billions of US dollars of sales, beneficial to industry and sometimes participating epilepsy centres, but have only slight benefit to an individual or society. Fraud and scientific misinformation is another dark side that is rarely mentioned.

The Burden of Drug-Resistant Epilepsy

Epilepsy that cannot be treated is called drug-resistant epilepsy. The improvement of seizure control in this situation is one of the most important unmet needs in the field of epilepsy. However, knowledge around this topic is incomplete or substandard. Definition is not even agreed. The criteria of the ILAE apply the term to any patient in whom at least two trials of adequately selected and dosed antiepileptic drugs have not brought sustained remission. This is a definition based on data which has suggested that failure of two drugs means that the chance of subsequent success is minimal. However, this quite clearly is not the case in large numbers of patients, and much depends on which drugs have been tried and on the characteristics of the epilepsy. Others have suggested that epilepsy should be considered drug resistant if treatment does not stop seizures for at least 12 months during the early years of therapy. This definition is based on an influential hospital-based observational study in which 36% of newly treated patients ended up with drug-resistant seizures, defined as not being seizure free for at least 1 year during the first 7 years since the start of epilepsy (2). If the definition included only frequent and severe seizures despite optimal treatment is used, only 5–10% of newly diagnosed patients are estimated to have drug-resistant seizures. A diagnosis of absolute drug resistance by other definitions requires failure of at least six antiepileptic drugs.

The mechanisms underlying drug resistance are still not understood, and not a single current hypothesis convincingly explains how drug resistance arises in human epilepsy. A new synthesis or conceptual breakthrough is needed. Interestingly, drug resistance is more common in those with a history of depression and in those with high frequencies of seizures before treatment onset, and these observations suggest that common neurobiological factors might underlie disease severity, psychiatric co-morbidity, and drug-resistant epilepsy. The absence of any clear idea about mechanisms, causes, or for that matter even definition, however, results in physicians having to make decisions in a fog of considerable uncertainty.

Whatever the mechanism, over one-third of people with epilepsy (over 20 million of the 65 million patients worldwide) at any one point in time are 'drug resistant'. As will be clear from preceding chapters, there are many possible drugs that can be tried. Antiepileptic drugs are often divided into the old (classic drugs) which were introduced into practice before 1989, and the new (novel drugs) which were introduced after this date. As mentioned earlier, though, there is no real evidence that the new drugs as a group are more effective than the old drugs as a group. Furthermore, about 50% of newly treated patients report at least one, mostly mild, adverse effect from proper treatment with the new as well as the older drugs (3). There is no compelling evidence that, as a group, the more recently approved drugs are better tolerated in terms of common but mild side effects than older ones. The serious and life-threatening drug reactions occur more commonly with older drugs, but fortunately are extremely rare (only around of 1 in 10 000 patients or less). The risk of malformations or cognitive problems in the offspring when taken during pregnancy (teratogenicity) is unknown with the newer drugs and varies also amongst the older drugs. Valproic acid is the drug which carries the greatest risk in in this regard (3). Taken as a group, the newer drugs also have less detrimental drug–drug interactions than older drugs, but there are exceptions to this general trend.

Another burden of drug-resistant epilepsy is the 20 times higher risk of premature mortality. Studies from developing countries normally report greater mortality than those from developed countries, probably partly due to more limited resources for epilepsy care, less medical training, and availability of treatment. Social and cultural differences are also of vital importance. It has been shown in the United States, for instance, that people with epilepsy from ethnic minorities do less well than white people. Death rates are substantially higher in patients with epilepsy who are not seizure free and in one large series, 55% of deaths were related to a seizure, and the causes included sudden unexplained death in epilepsy (SUDEP) in 38%, status epilepticus in 7%, and accidental drowning in 10%. The premature deaths that are not related to epilepsy were often due to the underlying disorder or to medical disease that developed after the onset of the epilepsy such as pneumonia (4).

Contributing to the dark side of epilepsy are many disorders that occur more commonly in people with epilepsy, and especially those with drug-resistant epilepsy, and these are sometimes known as 'co-morbidities'. The comorbid disorders include cardiac, gastrointestinal, and respiratory disorders, stroke, dementia, and migraine. Alzheimer's disease and migraine are not only more common in patients with epilepsy but are also risk factors for the development of epilepsy, suggesting shared disease mechanisms. The lifetime community-based prevalence of depression, suicidal ideation, and generalised anxiety disorder is twice as high in patients with epilepsy as in the general population. Depression and anxiety destroy quality of life and may cause an increased suicide rate. Psychogenic non-epileptic seizures or panic attacks may also be part of additional psychiatric co-morbidity. Psychiatric problems may lead to a poor response to the treatment of the epilepsy, whether by drugs or surgery, and may contribute to adverse effects when taking antiepileptic drugs.

Antiepileptic drugs such as phenobarbital, vigabatrin, topiramate, tiagabine, levetiracetam, and clobazam can cause or worsen depressive symptoms in patients with epilepsy. Stopping carbamazepine, valproate, lamotrigine, and pregabalin can cause depression because these antiepileptic drugs are mood stabilisers. Treatments for psychiatric disorders in patients with epilepsy are severely lacking which is another facet of the dark side of epilepsy for many patients. Current clinical experience suggests that carbamazepine, valproate, and lamotrigine cannot counteract established depression in patients with epilepsy. Although pregabalin is approved separately for epilepsy and generalised anxiety disorder, it has not been comprehensively studied as treatment for patients with epilepsy and comorbid psychiatric disorders. The ability of antidepressants to counteract depression in patients with epilepsy has not been properly assessed although there are some low-value studies suggesting that antidepressants may reduce seizures and depressive symptoms in patients with epilepsy and depression, but controlled trials are needed.

In developing countries, a further problem is the limitation to easy access to care. This is one reason for the astounding fact that the treatment gap, a measure of the proportion of patients with epilepsy who are untreated at any one time, is as high as 80–90% in many developing countries. This is even more distressing as epilepsy imposes a particularly large economic burden on patients and their families in rural and remote regions of the developing world and ironically it is the poorest countries which have the fewest publically funded health services. The stigmatisation and discrimination against patients adds further burden. Social isolation, emotional distress, dependence on family, poor employment opportunities, and personal injury add to the suffering of people with epilepsy. Because of the seriousness of the disorder and its psychosocial and other dimensions, it is worrying that epilepsy is often imperfectly diagnosed and managed, even in developed countries, and especially among low-income groups, and this is discussed further below.

In passing, we should also note that the burden of epilepsy can also be significant in those with rare seizures. Some patients have gaps lasting months and years between seizures but as the unpredictability of seizures, not knowing when the next will strike, is one of the most disturbing elements of having epilepsy, this applies as much to those who have occasional attacks as to those with very frequent seizures. Although uncertainty is an important constituent of life, most people except perhaps those with migraine, are only rarely exposed to so many attacks. Patients with few seizures share the same disadvantages of 'having epilepsy' (or as it has been called being epileptic) as those with more regular attacks. The best treatment strategy is also less clear-cut in such cases, and several questions arise. For instance, what is the best drug for rare seizures? Antiepileptic drug trials, for their own statistical reasons, prefer participants having many seizures, and there are none in those with less frequent attacks. Is it right to take drugs every day, to prevent an event which might occur only once or twice a year? Can this still be called epilepsy? There are no long-term studies of the natural history of epilepsy in those with rare seizures. Not knowing how their epilepsy will develop is another source of anxiety which undermines self-confidence.

Clinical Trials: What's Wrong With How We Assess Antiepileptic Drugs?

The fundamental 'unit' of epilepsy is the epileptic seizure. This is what might be called the minimum criterion of any definition and is of course what is targeted by drug and surgical treatment and documenting a 'change' in seizure frequency is at the heart of all therapy assessment. The 'seizure frequency' is usually recorded on a 'seizure diary', calendar, or notebooks and is a fundamental part of a routine clinic visit. Herein lies a problem. Increasingly, studies have shown that such methods are hopelessly inaccurate. Patients are sometime unaware that a seizure has occurred or, even if aware, forget to record it. Seizures occurring at night and unobtrusive seizures particularly are often missed. Objective studies using monitoring devices have consistently shown gross under-reporting of seizures in many instances. This is a bizarre situation, for the licensing of drugs is based almost entirely on these hopelessly inaccurate data—and the same applies to assessing surgery. A study from Bonn compared the patient's diary to seizure occurrence during video-EEG telemetry in 91 patients (5). A total of 582 partial seizures were recorded of which only 44% were recorded by the patient. Even major seizures were missed as were four out of five seizures at night. The authors concluded bluntly that 'patient seizure counts do not provide valid information' and it is difficult not to agree with this bleak statement. Others have made similar findings and the recent gold standard investigation by Mark Cook in Melbourne, using long-term monitoring with implanted electrodes, found that 8 out of 11 patients studied underestimated the real seizure rate by at least threefold (6). One patient, for instance, had 126 seizures recorded per month and considered that none had occurred, and another recorded a monthly seizure rate of 11/month when in fact the true figure was 102/month (7). The implications go far beyond routine practice, and the same data is used in clinical trials, questionnaires, and epidemiology. The scale of this problem is so large that doctors, authorities, and regulators have all failed to confront or even consider this, and in the rest of this section, issues of drug assessment are outlined which ignore this fundamental issue.

Both the classic older and the newer drugs are 'seizure suppressing' (i.e. not curative) and there is, as described above, not much difference in the strength of the suppressant effects between the older versus newer drugs as a group. One fundamental reason for this is that the strategies that have produced the older and newer drugs are similar. Simple seizure-provocation tests using the MES and PTZ have been instrumental in the identification of most antiepileptic drug candidates. This is what is known as an acute seizure test, and these have the advantages of technical simplicity and that large numbers of compounds can be screened. A major and perhaps fundamental flaw is that the seizures do not mirror epilepsy, simply because they are provoked and occur in 'normal', non-epileptic brains. This is why these animal tests are poor models of epilepsy. A second issue is that in these experiments, the older antiepileptic drugs provide complete seizure suppression and so do not allow the identification of new antiepileptic drug candidates with greater efficacy. The third flaw of the traditional approach to screening drugs using a small number of seizure models is that the process is likely to identify 'me-too' drugs and not those with completely different modes of action. More recently, large antiepileptic drug screening programmes in academia and industry have recognised these points and newer tests have been introduced which assess different actions. How predictive these newer tests are of human pharmacoresistant epilepsy remains unclear. It is a concern though that several potential compounds, for instance carisbamate, were highly effective in the new 6-Hz mouse test, for instance, but were not very effective in patients with pharmacoresistant partial seizures. Importantly, too, newer chronic seizure tests, such as the lamotrigine-resistant kindled rat, in which seizures are induced in animals with chronic brain alterations, have been recently included in the NINDS Epilepsy Therapy Screening Program, but none of the emerging tests, which often are misleading called models of therapy-resistant epilepsy, have been validated in predicting success in therapy-resistant patient populations. Whether the use of chronic experiments, such as kindling or in animals with spontaneous recurrent seizures, will lead to the identification of more effective antiepileptic treatments remains to be seen. Hopefully, this approach carries promise, particularly when testing hypothesis-driven, target-based strategies of drug development.

Other reasons exist for the failure to identify really distinctive drugs. Three strategies have been used in antiepileptic drug discovery: first, the random screening of newly synthesised compounds of diverse structural categories with as yet unknown mechanisms; second, the screening of structural variants of known antiepileptic drugs; and third, hypothesis-driven, target-based drug design. The first approach depends on luck and the second tends to produce 'me-too' drugs. The third is more intellectually promising, but in fact has identified only a few effective drugs, and none so far has been popular in clinical practice. Of course, much depends on whether the target mechanism is in fact truly central to the occurrence of seizures or the process of making a brain epileptic (the process is called epileptogenesis), or both, and in many instances in the past this has unfortunately proved not to be the case. The drugs derived by target-based drug design, at least to date, have been predicated on presumed mechanisms of seizure generation such as impaired GABAergic inhibition (vigabatrin or tiagabine) or increased glutamatergic excitation (perampanel), but the old reductionist (and simplistic) view that seizures or epilepsy are due to an imbalance between GABAergic inhibition and glutamatergic excitation ignores the complexity of the alterations within these neurotransmitter systems and neuronal systems. Target-based design crucially depends on the validity of the target, and most target theories turn out to be flawed. There is however hope and reason to believe that today's mechanisms will not fall by the wayside as others have done in the past. There is a measure of naivety amongst scientists who truly believe in the pre-eminence of their theories over others; and for the patient wanting a breakthrough treatment, at least for it seems that there is guarded reason for optimism in much of the current targeted-drug approach.

A common frustration among people with epilepsy and their physicians is the trial-and-error style of finding the best medication. A physician might ask a patient to start taking a common antiepileptic drug for a few months and see if it works. If it doesn't, they start over with a different drug which is often added to the medication. The fraught process can mean weeks of suffering and false hope for patients, but there seems to be no other way to do it. The reason may be that two people with identical focal seizures have different epilepsy mechanisms in their brains: one might have a problem with the GABAergic system, and the other with sodium channels. There's no way for physicians to know in advance, and no test which can indicate which drug is likely to be most effective. The downside for patients are suffering, time, and, for those paying for this random process, money. The situation is similar for other mental health disorders such as depression, anxiety, or attention deficit hyperactivity disorder. Several pharmaceutical companies recognise the problem and are analysing huge amounts of data, they call it big data, looking for 'biomarkers'—correlations which have some predictive power. Genetic testing, has been tried, and has proved helpful in guiding treatment in some cancers and rarer conditions such as cystic fibrosis. However, in epilepsy and in other psychiatric conditions, this search has to date proved fruitless and it is clear that genetic testing for identifying patients likely to respond better to any specific treatment still has a very long way to go, and the journey, at least currently looks bumpy to us. Another reason for the dismal situation we find ourselves in is that the regulatory trials have not been designed to assess the obvious question of patients whether a new drug had added value over standard drug treatment.

There are issues, with clinical trial designs, that may have contributed to the lack of progress in the discovery of more effective antiseizure drugs. The use of clinically irrelevant controls, such as placebo or substandard dosages of other antiepileptic drugs, rather than an existing gold standard treatment, prevents the identification of agents with improved effectiveness again standard treatment. Traditionally, the efficacy of new antiepileptic drugs is initially tested in placebo-controlled adjunctive therapy (add-on) trials. The primary outcome in epilepsy trials is typically the responder rate defined as the proportion of patients with 50% or greater reduction in seizure frequency during the treatment period compared to their baseline rate.

Efficacy is demonstrated when response to the active compound is superior to placebo. If factors exist that increase the placebo response it will be more difficult to detect the efficacy of a new antiepileptic drug. A major medical disadvantage of placebo is that several clinical features have been shown to influence the magnitude of the placebo response. Higher age at study entry improved the chances of having a placebo response of at least a 50% seizure reduction compared to baseline. A history of seven or more prior lifetime antiepileptic drugs compared to one to three prior lifetime antiepileptic drugs, a higher baseline seizure frequency, and prior epilepsy surgery all reduce the placebo response (7). A failure to control for these factors in trials of investigational antiepileptic drugs is a serious methodological flaw. Although the role of placebo to establish internal validity is appreciated, these important issues challenge the traditional position that placebo is a justifiable control for antiepileptic drug trials in epilepsy and raise interest in standard-of-care controls. Indeed, the potential for harnessing the power of a placebo is discussed further in Chapter 8.

In addition, ethical concerns exist with using placebo. Regulatory drug trials using placebo delay or deny proper treatment for participants. Furthermore, a recent study demonstrated an increased rate of unexplained sudden death in placebo arms of trials and this raises concerns about the safety of using placebo as a control (8).

Given the disadvantages of placebo, efforts are underway to de-emphasise its use in clinical trials of epilepsy. Novel add-on trial designs, such as the time to the nth seizure versus placebo in refractory epilepsy, minimise placebo exposure and give rapid answers about the efficacy of the treatment without insisting that non-responders stay in the clinical trial. In addition, and this may be a powerful incentive to avoid placebo, an expedited approval approach for breakthrough therapy is offered by the FDA. A FDA breakthrough approach is possible if preliminary clinical trial evidence is indicating that the drug may demonstrate substantial improvement over existing therapies on one or more clinically significant end points for a serious or life-threatening disease or condition. This new FDA programme is open to antiepileptic drugs and reinforces the need to include standard-of-care controls and clinically useful end points in early trials.

Another grave concern on the dark side of epilepsy is that placebo-controlled trials generate results of low clinical value. The conditions in which adjunctive therapy antiepileptic drug trials are designed and conducted have profoundly changed for the worse over the past decades. In the 1980s and 1990s when second-generation antiseizure drugs were developed, trials were conducted primarily in the United States or Western Europe using less than 15 sites, each of which enrolled and followed as many as 20 patients. A single monitoring organisation was often responsible for auditing all sites in the trial. Placebo response rates in subjects with partial seizures were relatively low, possibly because the epilepsy diagnoses and seizure classifications were correct. In addition, only approximately five antiseizure drugs were available for use 20 years ago, at least in the United States. Many subjects who agreed to enrol into trials had failed all the available drugs (9).

Today, large phase III trials require often a hundred or more clinical sites with each site enrolling as few as two patients. Trials are necessarily conducted in many centres and often internationally, in countries in several continents. This introduces variables which cannot be controlled for, and which risk obscuring scientific validity. The health resources available for baseline treatment can differ considerably, and patients entered into the studies can have a variety of comorbidities, treatment histories, and motivations. For logistical reasons, multiple monitoring organisations may be responsible for the auditing of these trials. Moreover, the clinical sites enrolling study participants are no longer exclusively specialised research institutions and trial investigators are often general neurologists rather than epilepsy experts. The ascertainment of eligible study participants is subject to high variability and misclassification may occur with patients without epilepsy or with a seizure type excluded from the study erroneously being recruited in the trials (9).

Current trial designs have also failed to acknowledge the heterogeneity of epilepsy and in particular in disease severity. It is well known that clinical features such as lifetime exposure to an increasing number of antiepileptic drugs are associated with a decreased likelihood of remission in patients with new-onset epilepsy, yet current trial designs do not stratify patients based on disease severity—for example, by the number of prior antiepileptic drugs the patients have been prescribed. The clinical trial designs used at present have led to the identification of many novel antiepileptic drugs, most were of similar, and indeed some of lesser, efficacy to older antiepileptic drugs.

Another major problem of current drug trials is that they consistently employ end points of low clinical value. A 50% reduction in seizures versus baseline is a measure of moderate clinical improvement and has been accepted by regulatory agencies worldwide as evidence for antiseizure efficacy of new antiepileptic drugs tested for add-on treatment of refractory, mostly partial, seizures. A recent meta-analysis of placebo-controlled trials has shown a difference of only 21% in favour of adjunctive new antiepileptic drugs over placebo for 50% seizure reduction (10). However, 50% reduction in seizures hardly improves quality of life in most patients. Unfortunately, the numbers of patients achieving freedom from seizures, which is the gold standard test for an antiepileptic drug for physicians, over that seen of placebo in these studies was only 6% (even in the short term) (10).

In most drug trials of epilepsy, the new drug is added to existing therapy. Although adjunctive treatment with modern antiepileptic drugs is standard care in refractory epilepsy, we know that adding another antiepileptic drug is often not a very effective strategy. This is not a new insight. As early as 1982, the results of a careful clinical observation in patients with refractory focal seizures suggested that the common practice of adding another drug in difficult-to-treat cases may need to be reconsidered until further evidence is presented that two drugs are more beneficial than one drug in the treatment of intractable epilepsy (11). A seizure reduction by more than 75% was seen in only 4 of 30 patients (13%) exposed to an additional second drug in the event of failure of optimum one-drug treatment. The remaining patients (87%) did not benefit from the second drug; in three patients the seizure frequency increased by more than 100% (11). Such benchmark studies in the early 1980s did not, however, lead to better trial design.

Despite the disappointing evidence, there is a persistent belief that many patients with epilepsy require concurrent treatment with more than one antiepileptic drug (which is called somewhat euphemistically rational polytherapy). However, there is not a shred of reliable evidence in human epilepsy (or in animals) that add-on treatment is more effective than monotherapy with the added compound. Despite their name, adjunctive regulatory trials cannot provide such evidence simply because they never test whether adding an antiepileptic drug is more effective than monotherapy with the antiepileptic drug that was added. In addition, no reliable information is available as to which drugs might work best in combination. One popular theory is that combining two drugs with different mechanisms of action might be particularly effective. Proponents of this idea tend to overlook the fact that there is scant clinical evidence for this belief except perhaps in relation to clinical situations in which there are pharmacokinetic interactions. Quantitative techniques such as isobolography can be used to compare the efficacy and side effects of antiepileptic drug combinations in animals. However, neither such methods nor antiepileptic drug mechanisms of action have yet proven useful in predicting clinical benefit in patients. Up to this day, antiepileptic drug choice in patients with epilepsy remains empirical.

Another type of study with remarkably low clinical value are the long-term follow-ups after clinical trials (sometimes called retention studies), yet the literature is swamped with them. They tend to offer inflated treatment effects not least because the studies are uncontrolled for placebo response, are prone to the statistical effect known as regression to the mean, and allow changes in the concomitant drug treatment to be made which make a nonsense of attribution of the observed effect to the experimental treatment. Furthermore, the populations are self-selected and potentially enriched as non-responding patients drop out. These studies are ignored by the regulatory authorities, but beloved by the pharmaceutical industry, and are heavily promoted at least partly it seems for commercial reasons.

Many antiepileptic drugs that are marketed for adjunctive treatment are subsequently tested in monotherapy trials in patients with either refractory or previously untreated epilepsy. Testing new antiepileptic drugs in monotherapy avoids the problem of lack of assessment in the presence of other medication, but other difficulties arise and some currently used monotherapy trials have clinically and ethically questionable designs. The favoured monotherapy development paradigm in Europe for new-onset epilepsy is the non-inferiority trial design, which establishes a present limit for the allowed poorer result in outcome between the test drug and a standard antiepileptic drug. The European Medicines Agency (EMA) accepts studies that demonstrate non-inferiority to an antiepileptic drug with established use as monotherapy. However, the FDA in the United States does not, because of justified concerns, elegantly expressed by Paul Leber, formerly with the FDA, who pointed out that both antiepileptic drugs could be equally ineffective. Monotherapy studies demonstrating superiority to placebo raise ethical concerns and non-inferiority studies identify poor or no better drugs but fail to identify added benefit. A conversion to monotherapy study design using a known effective agent administered at non-effective dose for many patients (technically known as low-dose active control, also referenced to in some studies as 'pseudo-placebo') was used in previous epilepsy studies but is incompatible with the Declaration of Helsinki and is no longer considered ethical by the epilepsy community.

These days, of course, a clinical trial is not just a scholarly affair, as many of us like to think, but is also a global, multibillion-dollar business enterprise, powered by the pharmaceutical and medical-device industries and for-profit clinical research organisations. The potential ethical problem today is not merely that these corporations have sufficient money to influence the directions of clinical research in universities which are often in poor financial condition. It is also that researchers themselves, particularly in developing countries or epilepsy centres anywhere with poor health resources, may be tempted by powerful financial incentives to pressure vulnerable subjects to enrol in studies, fudge diagnoses to recruit otherwise ineligible subjects, and keep subjects in studies even when they are doing poorly. These are unethical practices and that they go on is in no doubt, but the extent to which this happens is difficult to estimate. To be fair, the pharmaceutical industry has taken rigorous steps to safeguard the integrity of clinical trial data, and clinical research organisations are committed to monitor standards and documentation of study outcome and there is no evidence that they do not do a good job.

New antiepileptic drugs have not very substantially improved the treatment of patients with common seizure types (9). This begs the question of who is benefitting? One way to find the answer is to check the financial flows. Drug companies are in business to make money after all and have done so with several blockbuster antiepileptic drugs. New drugs are much more expensive than classical drugs such as carbamazepine, valproate, and ethosuximide and even more expensive than the older drugs such as phenobarbital and phenytoin which were introduced into the market in 1912 and 1938, respectively. If a company can convince physicians to prefer more expensive drugs, in the absence of compelling data that the new drugs are strikingly more effective for their patients, they are in business. One strategy is to ostracise valuable older drugs such as phenobarbital or phenytoin because of their side effects at high doses, doses which are not needed for successful therapy of most patients. At low daily doses these drugs are very effective and are well suited for people or economies with limited health resources when the alternative is having no treatment at all. Scare tactics have sometimes been used, showing people with side effects such as swollen gums while taking phenytoin or emphasising sleepiness on phenobarbital whereas this occurs mainly at doses of phenobarbital above what is usually needed for standard treatment. Of course, similar tactics are taken in other industries, notably the cosmetics or the fashion industry, but an important difference is that these items are chosen by the individual purchaser. The retail issue is that these drugs are not expensive enough to generate good margins compared to newer drugs which are much more profitable. In medicine, it is often the taxpayer who ends up paying for what is, in effect, often ineffective or unnecessary extravagance.

Low-Value Care

One of the darkest aspects of epilepsy is pervasive waste, which may be euphemistically called low-value care but that is really no-value care. Many patients, perhaps millions, undergo unnecessary blood tests including routine antiepileptic drug serum concentrations, serial EEGs when one or even none would be preferable, CT scans that are by now largely obsolete except for acute trauma care, MRIs, and taking too many antiepileptic drugs or much too high daily doses of antiepileptic drugs, that won't improve the epilepsy, might cause harm, and must cost many millions.

It may come as surprise but EEGs can be bad for patients. In fact, routine EEG recording is one of the most abused investigations in clinical medicine and is unquestionably responsible for great human suffering. The consequences of misread EEGs can be serious. They can lead to misdiagnosis, and studies have shown the shocking fact that 30% of patients previously diagnosed as having epilepsy do not in fact have epilepsy, and this mistaken diagnosis is often the result of misread EEGs. Subsequent normal EEGs do not cancel the previous abnormal one, and this makes an incorrect diagnosis difficult to undo, unless the 'abnormal' record itself is re-reviewed. The same does not apply to CT or MRI scanning. The reason is that the EEG is a functional test and findings genuinely vary over time.

Overdiagnosis can also occur due to over-medicalisation and this phenomenon is a very real one in epilepsy practice. As diagnostic technologies become more powerful, there is a tendency to identify ever-smaller 'abnormalities', to widen disease definitions, and to engender an enthusiasm for early detection. In other words, rather counterintuitively, overdiagnosis is a problem caused by too much medicine. The phenomenon of over-testing is made possible by all the new technologies we have for examining the blood and the brain. It is not easy for patients and doctors to recognise that tests and scans can be harmful. Why not have a thorough check and see if anything is abnormal? People are discovering why not. The United States is a country of 300 million people who annually undergo around 15 million nuclear medicine scans, 100 million CT and MRI scans, and almost 10 billion laboratory tests (10). Often, these are essentially fishing expeditions and since no one is perfectly 'normal', you tend to find a lot of fish. If you look closely and often enough, almost everyone will have a lab result that is a bit off, or an EEG or a MRI scan tracing that doesn't look quite right. Overdiagnosis is not necessarily misdiagnosis. It can also be the correct diagnosis of a disease that is so slight it is not going to cause discomfort or disability. An example is finding photosensitivity in an EEG or a small silent lesion in an MRI that is of no clinical relevance.

As pointed out nicely by Atul Gawande in his essay in *The New Yorker* on 'Overkill' in medicine (10), the patient is up against long odds. Doctors generally know more about the value of a given medical treatment than patients, who are not in a position easily to determine the quality of the advice they are getting. The forces, in Gawande's view, that have led to a global epidemic of over-testing, over-diagnosis, and over-treatment are easy to grasp. Doctors get paid for doing more, not less. They are more afraid of doing too little than of doing too much. And patients often feel the same way. They're likely to be grateful for the extra test done in the name of 'being thorough'—and then for the procedure to address what's found. Still, when it's your turn to sit across from a doctor, what are you going to fear more—the prospect of doing too little or of doing too much?

The misdiagnosis of epilepsy is an important aspect of the dark side of epilepsy. The misdiagnosis of epilepsy is particularly common and harmful in the emergency care room. In as many as one in six patients, the emergency room diagnosis of epileptic seizures turns out to be incorrect or missed (11). Epileptic seizures can be misdiagnosed and mistreated as psychiatric disorders or psychogenic non-epileptic seizures. Syncope is probably the commonest condition misdiagnosed as epilepsy, because of symptoms mistakenly thought to be confined to epilepsy, and this is of course a grave mistake.

Overtreatment is low- or even no-value care that may have serious consequences for patients with epilepsy (12). Quite frankly, as doctors, we are usually more concerned if we do too little than do too much. No patient with epilepsy should suffer more from the side effects of treatment than from the consequences of the underlying disease, and over-treatment is a constant risk, and in practice not uncommon. One major source of overtreatment is what has been called the 'therapeutic illusion', which is the unjustified enthusiasm for treatment on the part of both patients and doctors (13). Recommendations that might counteract the therapeutic illusion have been offered (13). The first is 'Before you conclude that a treatment was effective, look for other explanations'. And the second one is 'If you see evidence of success, look for evidence of failure' (13).

Overtreatment can occur in many forms. Long-term use (or continuation) of antiepileptic drug therapy in situations where it is not necessary (e.g. in children with uncomplicated, brief febrile seizures or in seizure-free patients) are obvious examples. The use of unnecessarily fast dose-escalation rates, which may expose the patient to potentially serious or severe side effects, or the prescription of unnecessarily high maintenance dosages are others. The latter may result from an inadequate understanding of dose–response relationships, from misinterpretation of serum drug concentrations (e.g. targeting concentrations within the 'range' in patients who are well controlled at lower concentrations), or, less often, from failure to recognise a paradoxical increase in seizure frequency as a sign of drug toxicity. The most common form of over-treatment, however, involves the unnecessary use of combination therapy (polypharmacy) in patients who could be treated optimally with a single drug.

Adverse effects associated with polypharmacy result from undesirable drug–drug interactions or from pharmacodynamic interactions leading to enhanced neurotoxicity (e.g. as seen in some patients given a combination of lamotrigine and carbamazepine). There is some evidence that some antiepileptic drug combinations (e.g. lamotrigine and valproic acid) might confer added value in some patients compared with either agent given alone, but this evidence is very weak, and the disadvantages of interactions are much more evident in routine clinical practice. In pregnancy, combinations, including those of valproate and lamotrigine, are associated more often with fetal malformations. Unless and until we better understand the complexities of drug combinations, single-drug therapy may avoid inadvertent over-treatment associated with polypharmacy.

Unfortunately, under-treatment of patients with uncontrolled epilepsy with suboptimal doses is also poor medicine. It is the normal clinical practice, in every patient with uncontrolled epilepsy, to incrementally increase the dose unless the patient has symptoms and signs of incipient side effects, and it has been shown that in as many as one in three patients presenting with uncontrolled seizures, increasing the dose led to seizure remission.

How can physicians get treatment right? Treatment of epilepsy is complicated and there are no simple solutions. However, therapy should be kept simple, unnecessary diagnostic or therapeutic interventions with an unfavourable risk–benefit balance should be avoided, combination therapies, especially with enzyme-inducing agents, should be avoided unless clearly necessary, but most importantly, therapy should be reviewed and kept under active surveillance with antennae tuned to problems both of under- and over-treatment—both are bad for patients and also society.

The Darker Side

There is no doubt that medical research has contributed immensely to societal well-being and to epilepsy. Medical research is rightly supported by public funding, industrial funding, tax breaks, and private funds. The high esteem of clinical research is, however, tarnished by concerns about the credibility of some clinical trials which have been criticised for lacking transparency and publishing favourable results only for the drug under investigation. Criticisms are made of conflicts of interest of researchers and of persistent commercial bias. Raw trial data are not publicly available and this limits the scrutiny of results by the public. Industry-independent confirmation of the outcome of large trials is also in practice prevented by the high cost. Critics claim that the publish-or-perish rule of the medical research industrial complex leads to many millions of publications that elude public scrutiny. They point out that even minor results are presented as a breakthrough based on enthusiastic press releases from the researchers or the university.

It is furthermore easy to introduce errors in clinical trial analysis. These include negligence and oversight and also a failure to employ adequate controls in clinical experiments. A clinical trial with all the exclusion and inclusion criteria is a highly complex model and does not and cannot mirror the clinical diversity of a treatment in clinical practice. The famous immunologist

Charles Weissmann is said to have posted the following warning on the door to his office: 'CAUTION: Do not enter this room without positive and negative controls'. Finally, blogs such as PubPeer or Retraction Watch will quickly publish results of post publication reviews to catch errors and fraud of researchers who cheat.

Physicians and the public rely on journals as unbiased and independent sources of information and to provide leadership to improve trust in medicine and the medical literature. Yet financial conflicts of interest have repeatedly eroded the credibility of both the medical profession and journals. As the Institute of Medicine explained in its 2009 report (14), a conflict of interest is 'a set of circumstances that creates a risk that professional judgment or actions regarding a primary interest will be unduly influenced by a secondary interest'. The key issue is that 'a conflict of interest exists whether or not a particular individual or institution is actually influenced by the secondary interest' (14) as it is not possible for editors and readers to know one way or the other. A related and controversial matter is whether editors should allow scientists who declare a conflict of interest to publish in their journal. Once conflict of interest has been declared, it is up to the perception of the reader whether to believe that the results or the interpretation are valid or not.

Fraud

The darkest side of all in the field of research, in epilepsy as in other medical areas, is the shadowy question of fraud. Scientists, not least because of their apparent stringency and quest for objectivity, are assumed to have high standards of transparency, and most do. However, this is sadly not always justified and there have been well-publicised examples of fraud which undermine trust in research, potentially damage patients, and obscure genuine advances. The cases uncovered are furthermore probably the tip of the iceberg, and the extent of deliberate fraud is unknown. Of course not all errors are due to fraud.

We both have encountered in our careers results that seem untrustworthy and researchers whose findings are never reproduced. There is a spectrum of dissemblance. Sometimes distorted findings are the result of unconscious bias rather than deliberate fraud, in other words poor science rather than dishonesty, and sometimes due to conscious data massaging (ignoring outliers or results which do not conform) and sometimes it is simply over-interpretation—hype and overenthusiasm with no malicious intent. Occasionally fraud is more deliberate but is justified by the thought that 'my theory must be right' or by the need to obtain more grant funding. Science is such big business now, that there is intense competition for grants and the all-persuasive pressure of the publish-or-perish culture. The medical researcher is often under intense pressure to perform and often burdened by oppressive and sometimes unnecessary regulations, bureaucracy, and management demands, and these increase the tendency to take short cuts. Whatever the motivation, it seems possible that there exists misinformation in the domain of scientific research (15). A detailed and scrupulous survey, reported in the journal *Nature*, found that 0.3% of researchers falsified data, 6% failed to present data that contradicted their results, 8% circumvented minor aspects of human subject requirements, 13% overlooked others' questionable interpretation or flawed data, and 16% changed study methodology in response to funding source pressure (16). It has also been estimated that approximately 10–20% of all research and development (R&D) funds are spent on questionable studies characterised by misrepresentation of data, inaccurate reporting, and fabrication of experimental results (17). A meta-analysis of studies similarly showed that 2% of all scientists admitted to having fabricated, falsified, or modified data, and over 33% admitted other questionable research practice (18).

In the latest field of genetics, we know of examples fuelled by a need to get grants and to fight for predominance in a competitive and disturbing university environment, and many go undetected but one example, recently uncovered, was a publication which claimed that four common subtypes of an inherited form of epilepsy were associated with three different mutations in a single gene coding for a chloride-gated ion channel. When the data were later re-examined for another genetics study, flagrant deceit was detected in the first study. A retraction letter was published but this was a full 6 years later. The editor of the journal congratulated the authors with the comment that 'This is probably the best example I've seen of authors correcting the record in a thorough way both through their own work and in collaboration with outside experts'. 'It's just a shame that it took them so long.' The most serious scientific misconduct, as occurred in this genetics study, is making up data to support a hypothesis. This happens occasionally, but the most common scientific misconduct is ignoring experimental data that does not support a hypothesis. Small 'glitches' occasionally produce contrary results, but, with experience, such random noise is recognisable and can safely be ignored. But what if 20% or 30% of your results contradict your hypothesis? It is patently unsafe to ignore this, but many scientists do. What can be done to limit fraud? We can start by ensuring that scientists, especially peer reviewers, are allowed to see the underlying data of a submitted manuscript, which researchers are typically reluctant to share. A federal Office of Research Integrity in the United States and a European institute of Research Integrity should be given funds and sufficient independence to investigate all major cases that come to its attention. We also need more research to determine how much how much deception there is and how to best combat it. The solution though cannot be entirely legislative, and science would benefit too from much more emphasis on an ethical culture and behaviour.

It is not only in the university setting that fraud exists, but perhaps less surprisingly it is prevalent also in the commercial environment in which the pharmaceutical industry has to function—highly competitive and one in which the dollar is king. The drug maker of one new antiepileptic drug recently agreed to pay more than $34 million and pleaded guilty to illegal promotion of the epilepsy drug for headaches and pain. The case is among scores of whistle-blower complaints that the US Justice Department has brought in recent years against pharmaceutical companies for illegal marketing of drugs including antiepileptic drugs. Physicians are free to use approved drugs for any purpose they see fit, but companies are prohibited from marketing drugs for off-label uses that have not been approved by the FDA as being safe and effective. The FDA approved the antiepileptic drug in 1999 to treat seizures in people with epilepsy and 5 years later, the company distributed posters claiming independent studies showed that the drug could prevent migraines. The posters did not disclose that the company had sponsored the studies, nor did they mention the fact that its own research had failed to show an effect on migraine as a result of which FDA approval of use in migraine was not sought. Despite this, the company's business plan allegedly showed migraine and other 'off-label' uses had much higher profit potential than those seen in epilepsy. Another company recently paid $400 million to resolve an investigation into alleged off-label promotion of another antiepileptic drug, as well as civil allegations relating to five other products. It pleaded guilty to misbranding through its illegal promotion. It was said to have offered financial inducements for doctors to prescribe the drugs, included payments for speaker programmes, advisory board membership, entertainment, travel, and meals to encourage doctors to prescribe the drugs. The company was alleged to have implemented an aggressive recruitment effort, designed to train up to thousands of physician speakers across the United States based, not on their experience or credentials as researchers, but their potential prescription-writing volume. Pharmaceutical company misdemeanour is tracked by a number of individuals and organisations. These include the website http://www.FiercePharma.com.

Sometimes, patients or their carers also mislead, another shadow in the epilepsy night. For instance, a husband from India recently complained in an Internet forum that after 1 month of marriage, 'I got to know that my wife has epilepsy (20–25 min attack) and that my in-laws hid this from me and my family. Now they are putting pressure on me and my family that accept the girl or else they will file the fake cases against me and my family. I don't want to continue this relationship and we are living separate from 7th march to till date. Is it possible to get this marriage nullified and is there any way to get divorce?' Intentionally under-reporting of seizures is a form of misrepresenting the truth to appease employers, to please the physician that the treatment works, or to convince relatives or oneself that epilepsy is a harmless disease. This is not altogether harmless as under-reporting may lead to injury when medication is not increased or to workplace injury or car accidents.

Perhaps the most unexpected form of misrepresenting the truth may be seen in parents of sick children such as in the following case. A prematurely born infant was admitted to hospital at the age of 6 months due to seizures which continued despite treatment even in an intensive care unit. Following 3 months of treatment and diagnostic work-up in three hospitals, intentional theophylline poisoning of the child by the mother was shown. Theophylline is a drug used to treat asthma. The seizures due to theophylline toxicity are well known in the literature. Non-accidental poisoning with theophylline occurred in the context of Munchausen syndrome (19). Munchausen syndrome by proxy is a relatively rare form of child abuse that involves the exaggeration or fabrication of illnesses or symptoms by a primary caretaker. Also known as 'medical child abuse', the syndrome was named after Baron von Münchhausen, as the name is spelled in German, an eighteenth-century German dignitary known for making up stories about his travels and experiences in order to get attention. 'By proxy' indicates that a parent or other adult is fabricating or exaggerating symptoms in a child, not in himself or herself. Munchausen syndrome by proxy is a symptom of psychiatric illness and requires treatment. Often, the cause is an abnormal need for attention and sympathy from doctors, nurses, and other professionals. Because the perpetrator appears to be so caring and attentive, often no one suspects any wrongdoing. Medical personnel often miss the diagnosis because the perpetrator is often very clever at manipulating and misleading physicians and nurses and it goes against the belief that parents and caregivers would never intentionally hurt their child.

References

1. **Sillanpää M, Schmidt D.** Natural history of treated childhood-onset epilepsy: prospective, long-term population-based study. *Brain* 2006; **129**:617–624.
2. **Kwan P, Brodie MJ.** Early identification of refractory epilepsy. *N Engl J Med* 2000; 342(5):314–319.
3. **Tomson T, Marson A, Boon P**, et al. Valproate in the treatment of epilepsy in girls and women of childbearing potential. *Epilepsia* 2015; 56(7):1006–1019.
4. **Sillanpää M, Shinnar S.** SUDEP and other causes of mortality in childhood-onset epilepsy. *Epilepsy Behav* 2013; 28:249–255.

5. **Hoppe C, Poepel A, Elger CE.** Epilepsy: accuracy of patient seizure counts. *Arch Neurol* 2007; **64**(11):1595–1599.
6. **Cook MJ, O'Brien TJ, Berkovic SF, et al.** Prediction of seizure likelihood with a long-term, implanted seizure advisory system in patients with drug-resistant epilepsy: a first-in-man study. *Lancet Neurol* 2013; **12**(6):563–571.
7. **Schmidt D, Beyenburg S, D'Souza J, Stavem K.** Clinical features associated with placebo response in refractory focal epilepsy. *Epilepsy Behav* 2013; **27**(2):393–398.
8. **Zaccara G, Giovannelli F, Schmidt D.** Placebo and nocebo responses in drug trials of epilepsy. *Epilepsy Behav* 2015; **43**:128–134.
9. **Löscher W, Schmidt D.** Modern antiepileptic drug development has failed to deliver: ways out of the current dilemma. *Epilepsia* 2011; **52**:657–678.
10. **Gawande A.** Overkill. *New Yorker* 2015; 11 May. http://www.newyorker.com/magazine/2015/05/11/overkill-atul-gawande
11. **Boesebeck F, Freermann S, Kellinghaus C, Evers S.** Misdiagnosis of epileptic and non-epileptic seizures in a neurological intensive care unit. *Acta Neurol Scand* 2010; **122**(3):189–195.
12. **Schmidt D.** Strategies to prevent overtreatment with antiepileptic drugs in patients with epilepsy. *Epilepsy Res* 2002; **52**:61–69.
13. **Casarett D.** The science of choosing wisely — overcoming the therapeutic illusion. *N Engl J Med* 2016; **374**;1203–1205.
14. **Institute of Medicine (US) Committee on Conflict of Interest in Medical Research, Education, and Practice.** *Conflict of Interest in Medical Research, Education, and Practice.* Washington, DC: National Academies Press; 2009.
15. **Broad WJ, Wade N.** *Betrayers of the Truth: Fraud and Deceit in the Halls of Science.* New York: Simon and Schuster; 1982.
16. **Martinson B, Anderson M, De Vries R.** Scientists behaving badly. *Nature* 2005; **435**:737–738.
17. **Glick L.** Scientific data audit—a key management tool. *Account Res* 1992; **2**(3):153–168.
18. **Fanelli D.** How many scientists fabricate and falsify research? A systematic review and meta-analysis of survey data. *PLoS One* 2009; **4**:e5738.
19. **Föll D, Debus O, Schmitt GM, Harms E, Zimmer KP.** [Life-threatening theophylline intoxication: a variant of Munchhausen syndrome by proxy]. *Klin Padiatr* 2003; **215**(2):86–89.

Chapter 7

Culs-de-Sac and Bureaucracies

The Culs-de-sac of Science: The Example of Epilepsy Aetiology

One of the important lessons of medical science, and no doubt all science, is that progress is erratic. Science is not, as sometimes portrayed, a process of linear advances with one discovery placed on top of another, and each relentlessly revealing the mysteries of nature. This is what might be called the *scientific fallacy* and, although reassuring to the gullible media and to the modern culture in which science has become the predominant discipline, it is wholly incorrect. Furthermore, science as much as any other human activity is dominated by fashion, and the idea of scientific 'objectivity' is largely spurious. The history of epilepsy provides a good example of the many wrong turnings taken in the name of science and the harm this has done to patients. False science is on epilepsy's dark side and the shadows continue to form to this day.

The theories of causation in epilepsy illustrate the point well, and here our point is that even in the scientific era of epilepsy, defined in this book as the years after 1860, the predominant theories of causation have often been embedded in societal trends and beliefs. This is a period marked intermittently by brilliant discovery on the one hand and on the other, some rather ridiculous propositions (1,2). The course of knowledge has meandered through fertile fields and stony culs-de-sac, and it is the capricious nature of this course which we emphasise here.

We have already seen how the modern scientific view of the condition became established by the work of John Hughlings Jackson, whose interesting view of causation is discussed further in Chapter 2. He felt that the cause of epilepsy was 'the instability of grey matter' and not the 'many pathological causes which lead to that instability' (3). In other words, he saw 'cause' as the 'causal mechanism', the molecular changes in the cerebral cortex that result in a seizure and not the downstream pathologies such as a tumour, trauma, infection, and so on. He was, furthermore, much more interested in the mechanisms of the 'instability' than in the downstream causes to which he gave little space in his voluminous writings. This was a remarkable intellectual insight which has not been given due credit and which has been taken up again only with the rise of molecular science. Another important principle of the nineteenth century is that the causation of epilepsy is almost always multifactorial. This was most elegantly demonstrated in William Lennox's charming 'stream and reservoir' analogy (published in 1960) in which Lennox emphasises that an epilepsy is the consequence of many different influences, some acquired, some congenital, and some genetic, and that the 'seizure threshold' similarly was the product of internal and external factors (Figures 7.1 and 7.2). There is a tendency today

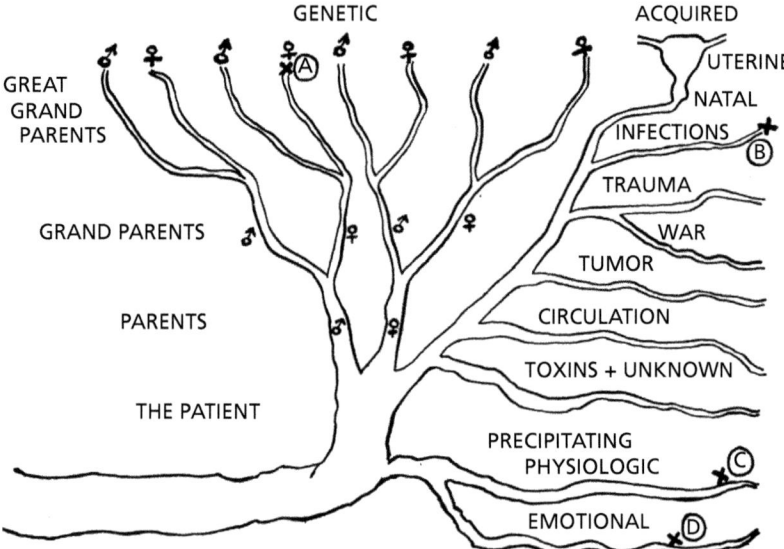

Figure 7.1 William Lennox published a famous pair of figures to illustrate his view on the multifactorial nature of causation in epilepsy. As he put it: 'The genetic watershed is represented … as three generations: parents, grandparents and great-grandparents [e.g. at A, a paternal grandmother has epilepsy]. A confluence of transmitted traits follows into (and through) the patient … In addition to these branching streams, there is an independent stream which rises in a lake (the uterus). The outlet is the birth canal and below that are contributing streams: infections [e.g. at B, a viral encephalitis], brain trauma from diverse sources, brain tumor, and circulatory disorders. This side stream enters the main stream at the patient level and combines with the genetic influences which had travelled through three generations to make him epileptic. There is then a third stream which enters below the confluence of the two main streams. This represents transient conditions which may precipitate certain seizures in a person already epileptic, or 'all set' to be. This evoking circumstance may be physiologic (say at C, hypoglycaemia) or emotional (say at D, a broken wedding-engagement)' (Lennox and Lennox, 1960).
Reproduced with permission from Lennox W and Lennox M. *Epilepsy and Related Disorders*, New York: Little, Brown & Co., Copyright © 2016 Lippincott, Williams and Wilkins.

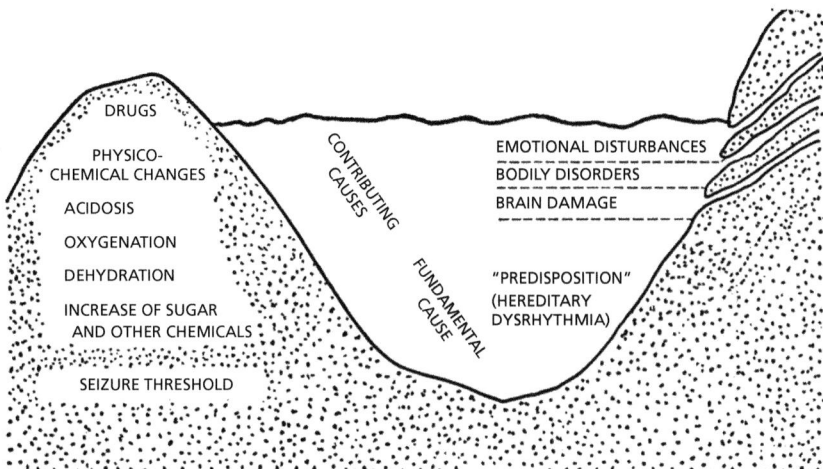

Figure 7.2 Lennox's causative factors of epilepsy seizures. In his words: 'Causes may be represented as the sources of a reservoir. At the bottom is the already present volume of water, which represents the person's predisposition, a fundamental cause. But the reservoir is supplied also by streams which represent the contributory conditions, such as lesions of the brain acquired since conception, certain disorders of bodily function and emotional disturbances. Periodic overflow of the bank represents a seizure' (Lennox and Lennox, 1960).
Reproduced with permission from Lennox W and Lennox M. *Epilepsy and Related Disorders*, New York: Little, Brown & Co., Copyright © 2016 Lippincott, Williams and Wilkins.

to overlook the multifactorial nature of causation of epilepsy but it is in fact a fundamental cornerstone of epilepsy theory.

One cul-de-sac from nineteenth-century science was the emphasis placed on heredity linked to the theory of degeneration (see Chapter 2). According to this theory, a wide range of conditions including epilepsy were inherited together. The conditions were thought of as manifestations of what was known as the 'neurological taint' (or sometimes known as the neurological trait or neuropathic trait) and included medical conditions such as insanity, psychiatric disorders, mental retardation, general paralysis of the insane, and locomotor ataxia, and also medico-social entities such as alcoholism, criminality, and sexual excess, including masturbation, or perversion. These conditions, it was believed, were inherited together and with a tendency for progressive degeneration over generations. The concept of the neurological trait was almost universally accepted by neurologists in the later years of the nineteenth and early years of the twentieth centuries. Linked to this was also the concept of atavism, related to Haeckel's theory of recapitulation, in which the degenerative process brings out atavistic characteristics. Epilepsy was seen as one such atavistic characteristic, in the downward degenerative spiral, occurring in around 20% of those with the neurological trait. Epilepsy was also linked to biological theories of criminality, ideas which now seem ridiculous but which had a profound influence on social theory and have had a lasting legacy in the medicalisation of aberrant behaviours and the concept that social behaviour has a biological basis. As outlined in Chapter 2, these themes led to stigmatisation and the rise of eugenics, which proved so catastrophic for people with epilepsy, but similar theories are still a focus of research albeit in altered form. There were other theories of causation of epilepsy, equally without any validity, but which were widely held in the early twentieth century. For instance, as part of the reflex theories of epilepsy, it was often considered that eyestrain led to epilepsy and many patients were subjected to tenotomies and pointless eyeglasses. Other reflexes thought to cause epilepsy included pain in limbs, pathology in ear or nose, or genital stimulation, and treatment suggested included surgical excision of traumatic peripheral nerve lesions, removal of a tight prepuce in boys, and of foreign bodies, adenoid growths, and polyps. All of this was fashionable illusion.

Another influential theory of causation was 'auto-intoxication'. It was believed that epilepsy was caused by internal toxins (not dissimilar to Galen's theory of humours), arising, for instance, from bowel, either through fermentation or from bacteria. This was part of a general public interest in toxins, both real and allegorical, which was a common cultural theme of the time. 'Scientific' studies using a sigmoidoscope or X-rays in 1910, for instance, showed 'acute angulation of the sigmoid colon' and 'impaction of the sigmoid' or 'coloptosis'. The results of animal experimentation were thought to confirm this, and inevitably surgical resection of the colon began to be practised. The psychiatrist Dr Henry Cotton, superintendent of Trenton State Hospital for the Mentally Handicapped in New Jersey, was a leading proponent of these ideas, and he carried out a very large programme of surgical therapy. In one 12-month period, 6472 dental extractions, 542 tonsillectomies, and 79 colon resections were performed under his direction and between 1918 and 1925, 2186 major operations was carried out. He had, by 1921, become a national celebrity, nationally renowned for his remarkable cure rates of epilepsy and psychosis by these means, and Trenton State Hospital was in 1921 declared by the President of the American Medical Association to be one of America's 'great institutions … a monument to the most advanced civilization' (2,4). This is a classic example of mistaken science, and there is not a shred of evidence to support the auto-intoxication theory. One shudders to consider the unnecessary pain and distress caused by the large number of destructive surgical procedures.

Another interesting interlude in the theories of causation of epilepsy relates to psychoanalysis. According to some psychiatrists in the 1920s, the predisposition to epilepsy was caused by egocentricity, supersensitiveness, emotional poverty, and an inherent defect of adaptability to normal life. The epileptic attack was viewed by others to be a reaction to escape the intolerable irritation and a regression to a primitive mentality comparable to that of infancy or intrauterine life. Smith Ely Jelliffe, who was the one of the leading American psychiatrists of his generation, considered epileptic attacks to represent a direct flight into infantile sexuality. Wilhelm Reich considered that seizures were repressed libido, and that the seizures were coital equivalents, and similar theories were held widely in psychoanalytical circles.[1] The psychoanalytical theories of causation of epilepsy were widely held right up to the 1940s.

Of course most of the above theories of causation now seem irrelevant at best and ridiculous at worst. The point of reiterating them is to demonstrate that medical orthodoxies of the time can be wrong, and that scientific theory is based to a significant extent on fashion—and there is no reason to believe that the same is not true today. A sceptical perspective is needed, not least given the torrent of hype and misinformation in the public as well as scientific media. It has been throughout history, and remains today, difficult to sort out the true advances from those which will prove culs-de-sac of history.

As the twentieth century has progressed, some discoveries in the study of causation of epilepsy have endured and become influential, and three in particular are worth recording as these represent our current lines of thought and also illustrate some common features in the pattern of history of science. First is the view that epilepsy is often due to a structural abnormality in the brain. This was recognised by the early neurosurgeons and neurologists but it was only with the advent of angiography and air encephalography that investigations in life could reveal hidden causes. These had a large impact as shown for instance in a paper by the American neurosurgeon Walter Dandy in 1932. He stated that: 'the writer is confident that there is now assembled from experimental, pathologic, clinical and surgical studies a sufficient number of unquestioned facts to place epilepsy unequivocally upon a pathologic instead of idiopathic basis … the fundamental conception that in every case of epilepsy there is a lesion of the brain can no longer admit of doubt' (6). Then in the 1970s and 1980s, the introduction of CT and then particularly MRI had a profound and far-reaching effect, to the extent that today we can compile with great precision lists of structural causes, and their characteristics, which are associated with epilepsy (and which are incidentally, very different lists to those of Dandy). There are on the periphery of this body of work uncertainties about what is truly 'pathological' and what is 'incidental' but in general the uncovering of structural causes has been one of the most truly important developments in epilepsy. Noteworthy is the fact that knowledge has advanced, not as a result of new epilepsy theory, but rather because of the application of new technology.

Although the core technologies of MRI (and CT) were without question paradigm shifts that changed the whole field of epilepsy, they have been followed by a plethora of increasingly elaborate and esoteric variations which have not been of lasting value. These are mainly in the field of 'post-processing' where computerised analysis and manipulation of the raw data has produced pictures and mathematical models—of the brain flattened, normalised, edge enhanced, pixelated, displayed in colour, displayed numerically, with enhanced contrast, and myriad other analyses. Many of these efforts have produced only a little of practical value either clinically or scientifically, and much of the research which occupies acres of published space has not endured. Their inconsequentiality to the field of causation in epilepsy resembles that of auto-intoxication or psychoanalysis. The application of EEG and MRI technology in epilepsy illustrates another notable feature of scientific discovery in medicine, and that is its non-linear 'stop–go' nature. A major technological advance is usually followed by a steep rising curve of clinical revelation, but after a few years the 'low hanging fruit' has been picked, and the curve flattens out with most subsequent work being of small incremental value only.

The second influential area is that of the 'idiopathic epilepsies'. These were called, in Jackson's time, the 'genuine epilepsies', and are the epilepsies in which there is no visible brain pathology or structural abnormality, at least at the macroscopic level. It was assumed in Jackson's time that these were largely genetic in origin, and the course of the history of eugenics, outlined in Chapter 2, is an example of the potential dangers of this assumption. In the era of modern molecular genetics, the genetic basis of most of the Mendelian inborn errors of metabolism has been elucidated and this has been a tremendous scientific achievement. However, these are relatively rare conditions, and the biggest challenge in epilepsy is the uncovering of the mechanisms of the idiopathic generalised and idiopathic partial epilepsies. These are very common conditions but are not inherited in any straightforward manner, and only very limited progress in understanding the mechanisms of causation has been made. Enormous 'gene hunts' have been conducted but have not turned up anything of great significance. The current view is that these conditions have a multifactorial basis, with genetic, developmental, and epigenetic inputs (much like Lennox's rivulets) and it seems very unlikely that there is a single genetic cause for these the most common of the epilepsies, or even any particular single gene which causes a significant degree of susceptibility. Brain development and the many factors influencing this (including the important influence of chance) may also be of crucial importance in the production of idiopathic epilepsy. Another interesting point about these conditions is that they are often liable to provocation by environmental factors, alcohol or lack of sleep, for instance.

Sometimes, the attacks only occur in the context, say, of lack of sleep and logically in these cases, lack of sleep is surely as much the 'cause' as is any predisposing genetic factor (albeit currently undiscovered). There is without doubt an insufficient current focus on provoking factors (in contrast to Jacksonian times, when their importance was perhaps overestimated) and the mechanisms by which they exert their effect.

The third area in which knowledge has truly advanced in relation to the causation of epilepsy is the field of molecular biology. This has focused on what Jackson thought was the real 'cause' of the condition, the molecular mechanisms at the level of the neuron. In the past 30 years there has been a true revolution in this field, with great advances in understanding of membranes, ion channels, neurotransmission, synaptic and axonal functioning, signalling, biochemistry, and single-cell physiology. Less advanced, but the focus of much interest, is molecular research into the more macro aspects of neuronal networks and systems. All this activity has led to very important insights into the mechanisms of epilepsy and there is much to celebrate in what has been achieved. However, it is important to retain perspective and a large part of this research, like much of the clinical work mentioned above, has proved not to have any long-term value. In part this is possibly due to the fact that the animal models which are used in experiments are often not very relevant to the human condition, and there is much debate about which are the best and most appropriate models (the old adage that 'the best model of a cat is a cat' still holds true). We are not experimental scientists and not in a position to express much of an opinion about this, but it seems clear from looking back at the published experimental work of 10 or 20 years ago, how little of it seems pertinent today. It raises interesting questions about whether medical research should be more focused, or whether an occasional important discovery can germinate only in the soil of irrelevant research. There has been one study looking at the extent to which clinical research publications are of enduring value. A methodology was developed using four different domains, and 300 papers published in 1981, 1991, and 2001 were assessed for their value 10 or more years later. It was found that 71% of the papers were categorised as having 'no enduring value' and only 4% as having 'high enduring value'. The 'no-value' papers typically reported something that was unimportant, not novel, or had significant methodological flaws (7).

It is interesting, too, to muse on the fact that there are whole areas of medical research in epilepsy which have resulted in little of lasting benefit to patients. In addition to psychoanalysis and theories of auto-intoxication mentioned above, and the many useless therapies and even surgical operations carried out for epilepsy in the modern era (see Box 7.1), one can speculate also about

> **Box 7.1 Some of the largely ineffective surgical procedures used to cure epilepsy 1860–1920**
>
> - Trepanation/trephination
> - Carotid artery occlusion
> - Bilateral vertebral artery occlusion
> - Cervical sympathectomy
> - Castration
> - Circumcision/removal of tight prepuce
> - Hysterectomy
> - Oophorectomy
> - Adrenalectomy
> - Dural splitting
> - Colectomy and other bowel resections
> - Arterialisation of internal jugular vein
> - Excision of painful peripheral nerve lesions
> - Adenoid and nasal polyp removal.

the limited value of some investigatory modalities such as isotope scanning, magneto-encephalography, or transcranial magnetic stimulation. There are two particular contemporary research areas, however, which have attracted the greatest adverse criticism, and these are those of functional brain imaging (fMRI) and some aspects of neurogenetics. Ray Tallis, in his book *Aping Mankind* (8), refers to these as neuromania and Darwinitis, and provides a withering attack on the kind of science which claims that it has discovered a 'gene for' kindness, a 'brain region for' taking out sub-prime mortgages, or experiments that 'prove' hard determinism or the universal selfishness of humanity. Tallis's greatest attack though is aimed at the use or rather misuse of fMRI in identifying brain areas—a sort of facile localisationism and the exaggerated claims made about the role of mirror neurons in empathy, brain scans in criminal responsibility, the temporal lobe in spirituality, and so on. A similar disparagement is found in the recent book *Genes, Cells and Brains* by the distinguished biologist Steven Rose and sociologist Hilary Rose (9), subtitled ironically *The Promethean Promises of the New Biology*. These technologies have been widely used to investigate cerebral function in epilepsy, and if Tallis is right it is difficult not to believe that these whole scientific areas will not suffer the fate of psychoanalysis. Both are popular in the public mind, both are spectacular (and MRI has the advantage of the production of attractive colour pictures), but both are in Tallis's view, and that of many others, almost entirely spurious.

Severe criticisms have also been levelled at the statistical basis of many studies in the field of neuroscience, including epilepsy. A leading critic in this area is John Ioannidis, Professor of Health Research and Policy at Stanford University. His 2005 paper 'Why Most Published Research Findings Are False' (10) is the most downloaded technical paper from the journal *PLOS Medicine* and its premise is that many medical research findings are flawed because of poor methodology and a poor statistical basis. Ioannidis analysed '49 of the most highly regarded research findings in medicine over the previous 13 years' and compared the 45 studies that claimed to have uncovered effective interventions with data from subsequent studies with larger sample sizes: 7 (16%) of the studies were contradicted, in 7 (16%) the effects were smaller than in the initial study, and 20 (44%) were replicated (and 11 (24%) remained largely unchallenged). This is not a good record, and he and others have raised increasingly convincing voices about the poor quality of research and the impact of commercial and societal influences on neuroscience[2].

The Bureaucracies of Epilepsy: The Medical Journal

One of the astounding bureaucracies of modern epilepsy is the 'medical journal'. The first scientific journal, the *Philosophical Transactions of the Royal Society*, was published in 1665 in London, and the first medical journal was *The Lancet* published from 1823. Initially the journals were ridiculed but have since become an indispensable feature of the scientific landscape. The speed of knowledge transfer, because of the system of journals, is extraordinary. We are always amazed at how quickly and efficiency information can be disseminated across the world. Of course with the rise of the Internet, this would now be possible without a 'journal' but the journal system is now so well entrenched, and the system so efficient, that it remains a leading method.

The phenomenal growth in the number of science, technology, and medicine (STM) journals is one of the striking features of modern academia. In 2008, there were more than 25 000 such periodicals, with 1.5 million papers published and 1.2 million authors publishing each year. The STM journal publishing industry has also become big business with an annual turnover in 2008 of $7.7 billion, and huge profits. This was partly due to the migration of the journals online, reducing costs and increasing readership, and the business model for journals has become so good that profits have soared. Richard

Smith, former editor of *The BMJ*, reported that in 2005 the annual turnover of Reed Elsevier, the biggest science and medicine publisher with 1800 journals, was £5166 million and the adjusted operating profit was £1142 million (15). It has been said 'All publishing is theft' and certainly a greater than 20% profit on annual turnover is a handsome return. Consider further that the articles are given to the journal for free (or nowadays, authors even pay), reviewers are asked to review without remuneration, and for many journals, such as *Epilepsia*, the editors are not paid despite devoting many hours to the task. Publishers meet the costs of technical editing (if any is offered) and design, but these are really possible at minimal cost. Distribution in the digital age has also become very cheap, via online platforms, and the print editions or journals are rapidly disappearing. Publishers market their journals largely electronically, and access is available online for individual subscribers, institutions, and libraries. The library subscriptions are very expensive but it is difficult to get information about the exact cost of any individual journal subscription, as this is obscured by the practice of selling bundles of journals together and selling the bundle, and there is also a myriad of individual negotiations. Where data is available, the costs of the journals can be extraordinarily high, and one notorious example was the Elsevier's journal *Brain Research* which cost \$23 617 for a 1-year library subscription. The Internet has created a business model which is astonishingly favourable to publishers, and in the field of epilepsy, for instance, *Epilepsia* only started to make a profit in 1989 (80 years after its foundation), when online publishing began, and it now nets some million dollars a year.

The journals are valuable assets. Many are owned by their publishers, but others by a learned society which gives the journal a captive audience, some respectability, and is considered often to be a sign of quality. *Epilepsia*, the most prestigious clinical journal in the field of epilepsy, for instance, is owned by the ILAE (Figure 7.3). The ILAE contracts all aspects of the management of the journal to its publishers who in return pay upwards of \$1 million to the ILAE annually for the privilege of publishing and running the journal, and one presumes, making a profit in the process. This is easy money for ILAE, and you might feel this is a win–win situation for epilepsy and the publisher, but of course it is at the expense of the subscribers and libraries which are often funded from the public purse. Furthermore, the value is retained by restricting access to the papers and this is discussed further below.

Epilepsia was the first journal devoted to epilepsy. It was published first in 1909, and after two early interruptions, has been in continuous publication since 1959 (16). In the field of epilepsy, *Epilepsia*'s monopoly ended in 1985, with the inauguration of the journal *Epilepsy Research*, then followed in 1988

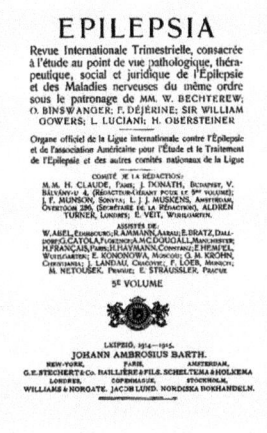
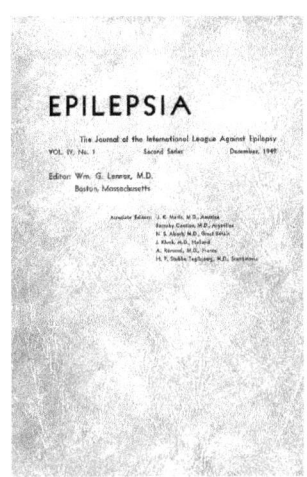
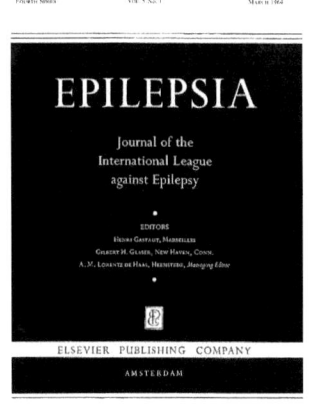
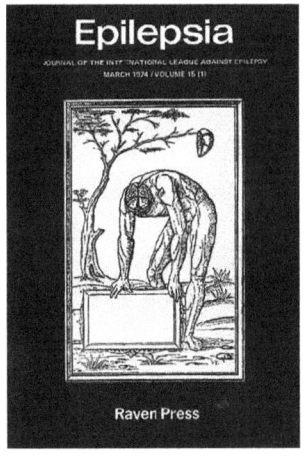
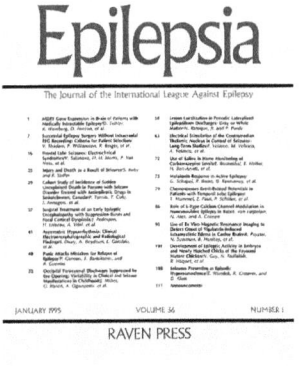
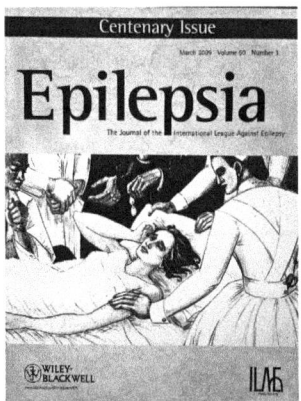

Figure 7.3 Covers of *Epilepsia* from (clockwise from top left) 1914, 1949, 1974, 2009, 1995, and 1964.
Reproduced with permission from The International League Against Epilepsy and John Wiley and Sons, Copyright © 2016 The International League Against Epilepsy.

by *Journal of Epilepsy, Seizure* in 1991, *Epileptic Disorders* in 1998, and *Epilepsy and Behavior* in 2000. The journals also increased in size and between 1985 and 2005, for instance, the number of pages annually in *Epilepsia* increased from just over 500 to well over 2000 (Figure 7.4). Another trend in recent years is for journals to become more focused. In 2011, it was proposed by the then *Epilepsia* editors that, to enhance the quality of *Epilepsia*, the ILAE should both launch an additional online open-access sister journal and also take over the ownership of *Epileptic Disorders* and convert this into an ILAE educational journal. These would, it was argued, allow *Epilepsia* to focus on its core mission, which was to publish high-quality scientific papers of high impact, by offering others ILAE forums for other types of paper. Although this proposal was turned down initially by the ILAE executive, the decision was reversed and in 2014 ILAE acquired *Epileptic Disorders* and in 2016 inaugurated a new online open journal (*Epilepsia Open*). Both are instructive demonstrations of the changing publishing landscape.

Since 2000, the growth of the worldwide web has resulted in an even greater explosion in the number of journals. It is quite possible, for an energetic young entrepreneur, to set up an entirely online journal, with almost no capital outlay, working for a few hours a week in their back room in any village of the world, and this is now exactly what happens. The number of scientific journals has

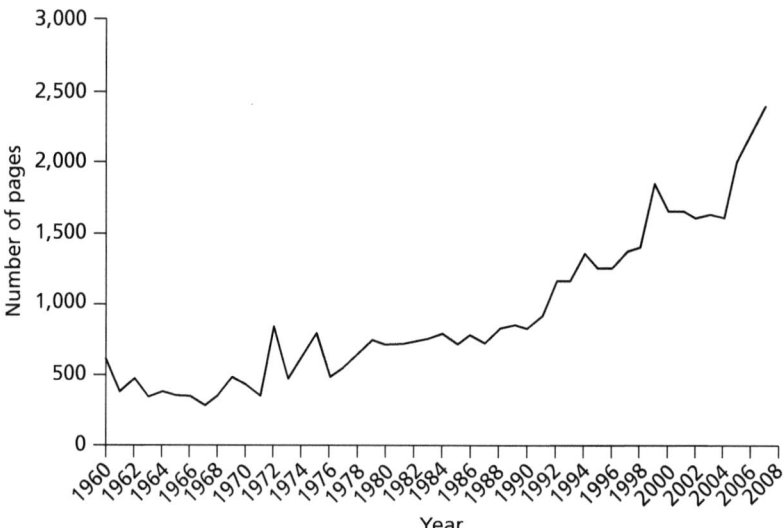

Figure 7.4 The growth in number of pages in *Epilepsia*.
Source: data from Wiley Online Library: *Epilepsia*, http://onlinelibrary.wiley.com/journal/10.1111/(ISSN)1528-1167, accessed 01 Oct. 2015.

risen from 3621 in 2001 to 5022 in 2011, and there are countless minor journals in the field of epilepsy flooding the email inboxes of doctors and institutions, hawking their wares, asking for reviewers, inviting random academics on to their editorial boards, and pimping for papers.

It is this good for epilepsy? At first glance, one might argue that the increase in the volume of papers might be good as the rapid and easy dissemination of good ideas and of sound medical science can only be beneficial to the patient. However, in practice, this is not how things are working out. Although there has been in the last 20 years a significant increase in the amount of research carried out in the field of epilepsy, the increased availability of publishing outlets has made it much easier to get work published, and as a result, poorer work which would not previously have passed muster, is now able to be published. The increase in the number of journal has without question reduced the overall quality of the published science. There has also developed an increasing tendency to publish and republish the same ideas, to salami-slice data into several publications, to publish review after review after review, to publish scientifically and methodologically flawed results, and to report trivial findings of less and less value. The academic world is now awash with inconsequential and often pointless papers; a veritable barrage of white noise, the scientific value of which is minimal. Let's hope that we are wrong with our bleak outlook.

Some research publication is so substandard that it seems to us that the primary reason cannot be communication of new knowledge, which after all should be what a journal is for, but for such purposes as enhancing an author's CV, a tendency exacerbated by the routine use of publication metrics in university promotion and the award of new grants. Publishers have seen the potential for easy profits from starting new journals, and have to an extent encouraged poor research by providing increasing numbers of journals to place the research. It is no exaggeration to say that any paper, no matter how bad it is, is likely to find publication somewhere, and as a result the medical literature is now bulging with low-value reports, and this mass of poor papers carries the risk of obscuring important papers or burying important findings. We live in a world where there is information overload in many areas, and it seems to us important that a more responsible attitude should be taken to conveying medical research information.

The challenge now is not to get a paper published, but to sift an article of real value or novelty from this scientific wreckage, and this has not escaped the attention of the academic community. A first and obvious response is to grade 'journals' and then use this grading to provide some sort of quality measure of the papers published. A variety of metrics have arisen, of which the most widely known is the so-called journal impact factor (IF for short). This is calculated by measuring how often papers in the journal are cited in other research papers, over a specific period of time. Many outside the field of science cannot believe that a system has been devised which logs the citations of individual papers in other papers, but as all is now electronic and we live in a world of big data, this is not as difficult as it might seem. The premise behind this is that the more often a paper is cited, the better or more valuable the paper must be. This of course is a crude measure and has inevitably led to gaming which has in turn had a distorting effect on the type of papers published. There is a sometimes an unseemly scramble for academics to get their names on papers which are likely to be well cited, and more senior a person, the more freewheeling seems to occur. Reviews flourish in this environment too, as it is easier (and lazier) to cite a review than the original research. The editors of some journals even ask the authors to cite articles in their own journal, in an effort to increase the IF. The real quality of a journal depends on the editor ensuring that decisions about the choice of papers to publish are based on the aims, nature, and mission of the journal, and not on metrics, but there is a distressing tendency nowadays for editors to select papers on the basis of IF. In our opinion, this will ultimately erode rather than enhance a journal's reputation, but it is a widespread practice. Of course, having said this, some objective system of grading the true worth of a paper is needed.

The validity of a publication relies on high-quality peer review. The process of peer review is at the heart of all journal publishing and is overseen by the editors, who choose appropriate people to comment anonymously on a submitted paper, and who then make a decision on publication on the basis of the review. There are manifold problems with this system, but no one can suggest a better one. For it to work effectively, the editors need to keep a very careful eye on the process and this seldom happens. Publishers increasingly ask random reviewers (our email boxes are full of such requests) and no doubt too keep databases (which some probably sell commercially) of reviewers and their interests. The explosion in the number of journals has led to peer-review exhaustion, and it has become increasingly difficult to find suitable persons who are prepared to take the time (often several hours) to review a paper thoroughly and to issue a report. Reviews are now more superficial than in the past, and can be mired in politics. Studies have shown that the agreement between two reviewers is often barely better than chance, and some argue that the process is a total lottery. There is no doubt some truth in this. However, when good reviewers are chosen and sensible overview is provided by the editors it can be a very successful form of effective oversight. In the field of epilepsy, though, which is relatively small, our experience as editors is that sometimes reviews are based on personal feelings and these have to be sifted. We have come across reviews that start 'This is as bad as it gets' or 'The understanding of genetics is no better than a high school student' and when one sees these, one knows the reviewer and the review will be inevitably partisan. An equal problem is that of superficiality, and if the reviews are carried out with insufficient thought, the result will be shoddy publishing and an unreliable published literature—and for many journals, some critics believe, this is already the reality.

Another consequence of the increase in papers and reviewer fatigue is the risk of undetected fraud. This is a shady area which is difficult to evaluate. However, anecdotal evidence suggests it is indeed on the increase. There are some authors whose data never seem to be confirmed and whose results seem too good or too unlikely to be true. We can think of several examples, and it is difficult not to believe that the data must therefore be flawed. Where findings are produced by individuals with much to gain from positive results (grant money, promotion, etc.), the temptation to fudge results, ignore outliers, or massage data may be, for some, irresistible. This seems a particular problem where big data is involved, and the fields of medical genetics, epidemiology, and treatment trials seem to be particularly at risk.

Authorship of papers is another difficult area. Increasingly, papers in epilepsy include multiple authors some of whom had very little to do with the study. The head of department or other senior figures often are added as a matter of course. This is a very poor practice, which continues despite well-publicised codes of practice for 'authorship'.[3] The order of authors listed on a paper is another common source of conflict in the competitive university environments—and we can think of striking examples of devious and poor behaviour of individuals in epilepsy research groups (often senior) insisting unreasonably that they should occupy the first or last berths on the lists of authors of papers which they had in fact very little to do with.

All these behaviours are fuelled by the fact that in recent decades, university and hospital promotions have come to depend to a great extent on an individual's publication record. An interesting statistic would be to quantify the increase in numbers of publications on CVs today compared to those from 20 years ago. We would guess this has tripled, and it is now not uncommon for a leading academic to have 600 or more papers to his or her name. This is a ridiculous situation and scrutiny of the papers shows how insubstantial some of the content is and often how little is an individual's true contribution.

A force ten storm raging in the turbulent landscape of medical publishing now concerns 'access'. In the traditional model, profits were made by publishers by selling access via subscriptions to individuals, libraries, and institutions.

This model has guaranteed a good return, and by raising prices, some publishers have made very large profits. Since the 1950s, there had been some pressure to allow published research to be made freely available to the public (i.e. non-journal subscribers) but this initially lead nowhere. However, in the last two decades, the 'open access' movement has gathered momentum, largely in response to growing disquiet over excessive profits of the publishing companies. In 2002, the 'Budapest Open Access Initiative' was launched. This was followed (with geographical rectitude) by the 'Berlin Declaration on Open Access to Knowledge in the Sciences and Humanities' and the 'Bethesda Statement of Open Access', and wholly open access journals began to be published. The US and UK government funding agencies, the Wellcome Trust, and others weighed in and demanded that the results of their publicly funded research should be available to the public. UK universities were then asked to ensure that academic articles submitted as part of the assessment for public funds (the Research Assessment Exercise) should be made available on university websites ('institutional repositories'). The movement has gathered an irresistible momentum, and the big medical publishers who were initially dismissive have scrambled to find a formula which allows profits still to be made in an environment when research papers are rapidly becoming free to all readers. One solution has been to make authors pay for submissions, and so we now have the unsavory situation where authors or their institutions are paying publishers to process their work (usually a fee of $2000–$3000 for a published article in the field of epilepsy) so that the publishers' margins can be protected. This of course is only worthwhile if it is considered that the journals add sufficient value, as the alternative course would be to simply publish a paper oneself on a university or personal website which is an option increasingly followed.

Key to access is a system of indexing to enable web-users to find a relevant research paper. Traditionally, searches are done via Medline (PubMed) or some such system which do not include university repositories or self-published articles. However, increasingly researchers are turning to search engines like Google, which are more powerful and quicker, and where repositories and self-published articles will appear. Self-publication though can have no peer review and indeed no review of any sort, and it is this which will probably ensure a future for the medical publishers. However, as the plethora of online journals of very dubious quality multiplies, and as the traditional journals find it harder and harder to conduct high-quality peer review, the distinction between the quality-controlled (peer-reviewed journal articles) and the non-quality-controlled (including self-published articles) is increasingly blurred.

The impression gained from this litany of problems may be too negative. It should not be forgotten that almost all genuine scientific advances are communicated via journal publication and the system has remarkable scope and reach. The rapid spreading of scientific information is indeed a triumph of human endeavour and has been a major achievement of global academia. Nevertheless, with the advent of the Internet and the irresponsible rise in the number of journals fuelled by the profit motive, the once-tranquil waters of traditional publishing are being stirred up in a whirlpool of uncertainly. What will happen to the epilepsy journals is not clear. It is likely they will not sink, but in surviving, the shape of their rigging is certain to be changed.

The Professional Bureaucracies of Epilepsy

Another interesting bureaucracy which arose in the twentieth century is that of the professional association—usually a grouping of doctors, forming a non-profit organisation to promote their field of medicine. These were initially almost invariably philanthropic endeavours, but as they have succeeded, some have become progressively globalised, and as they have grown, more commercialised. For some, their financial security has become dependent on the pharmaceutical industry. The role of professional organisations in society has also slowly changed over the course of the twentieth century, and the story of the ILAE provides an example of the sort of changes that have occurred in many different organisations.

The ILAE is most important professional association in the field of epilepsy, and one of the most important in neurology.[4] It was founded in 1909 in Budapest. At the time, it was comprised of individual members and not country chapters and was a small, mainly European organisation with, in 1911 for instance, 106 members. The organisation ceased activities in 1914 at the onset of the First World War, and was restarted in 1935 at a meeting in Lingfield in England. It then took the form of a federation of three chapters, Great Britain, the United States, and Scandinavia, and appointed an American President, because, as it was said, an American was 'uninvolved with the politics of Europe, which had proved so disastrous'. In 1939, the activities ceased again, but the ILAE was kept alive by its American chapter, and was again reconstituted in 1947. At the first post-war meeting in 1949, there were nine official national chapters, from Europe, North and South America. Japan joined in 1953 as the sole Asian country. Over the next three decades the organisation grew slowly in size and importance, and by 1987 there were 30 chapters. Since then there has been a rapid increase, and today there are chapters in 104 countries with over 16 000 individual members of the national chapters.

The two core functions of the ILAE have been, since its inception, the holding of congresses and the publication of an epilepsy journal *Epilepsia* (and now also *Epilepsia Open* and *Epileptic Disorders*). The conferences were initially held annually until the First World War, and since 1946, a continuous series of international congresses have taken place initially every 4 years and now biennially. These were, until 1978, attached to the congresses of the larger international neurology and neurophysiology organisations, but since then have been stand-alone. Until 1973, the meetings were short (1 day until 1973) but currently last for 4-5 days with multiple parallel sessions. At its first meeting, fewer than 50 people attended, but now routinely 2000 or more are expected. In addition to these international congresses, since 1994, regional congresses have also been held biennially in alternate years to the international congress. The European congresses were the first and are the biggest, attracting in recent times between 3000 and 5000 delegates. National meetings were also inaugurated in member countries in the mid 1930s, and an annual national meeting is now a prominent feature of ILAE affiliation. These meetings provide a vital function, keeping the life-blood of professional epilepsy circulating. Clinicians and researchers meet, findings are presented, and delegates are updated and kept abreast of recent developments. More than all of these, though, they provide a forum for networking and personal interaction—and it is this function alone which cannot be reproduced by the journals or online communication. The congresses are not perfect. They are expensive, mired in parish pump politics, and overshadowed by the looming presence of big pharma and commercialisation; nevertheless, the field would have advanced far less without them.

The second core function of the league is the publication of its scientific journal, *Epilepsia*. This has a complex history, appearing in four series: series I—1909-1914/15, series II—1937-1950, series III—1952-1956, and series IV—1959/60 to the present day. The first series was primarily a scientific enterprise, and published interesting and important papers, as well as reports of ILAE activities and critical abstracts of epilepsy publications elsewhere. When the second series was launched, the ILAE executive decided that the publication of scientific papers should not be the main focus, but that instead *Epilepsia* should contain abstracts of the scientific literature from elsewhere and act as a record of ILAE activity, turning it therefore more into a newsletter than a scientific journal. There were marked disagreements about whether the third series should continue along the same line or be more scientific, and a hybrid system was settled upon which was not a success. At the launch of the fourth series, the emphasis was again placed on publishing 'informed, original and critical studies' covering all fields of epilepsy research (18). Until 1989, the journal required ILAE funds to support it, since then, as discussed earlier, scientific journals have become profitable. The journal was published in full colour for the first time in 2007, and in that year, too, digital copies of the entire print run from 1909 became available online. The financial turn-around of the journal was due to the favourable business model discussed above. The large multinational pharmaceutical companies also contributed by routinely buying reprints and commissioning supplements as part of their marketing efforts.

In addition to its congresses and journal, the ILAE also has created a series of 'commissions' and 'taskforces'. The first, was the Commission on Classification and Terminology, established in 1963, and this commission formulated the 1969/1970 ILAE Classification of Seizure Type, discussed in Chapter 1, which is perhaps the most enduring and influential of all ILAE constructions. Tagging the classification with the ILAE name was a publicity coup, and it is probably no exaggeration to say that this single manoeuvre did more than any other to promote the ILAE and catapult the organisation into the top spot in the world of epilepsy. In 1969, the Commission on Antiepileptic Drugs became the second ILAE commission, and this too exerted a major influence on regulators and on industry, and was responsible in large part in formulating the structure of antiepileptic drug assessment. Inspired by the successes of the two commissions, in the 1980s, a range of other commissions and taskforces were put in place, each charged with different aspects of epilepsy work. With some exceptions, these have been, in our opinion, generally less fruitful, and some of their reports of less enduring value (Figure 7.5).

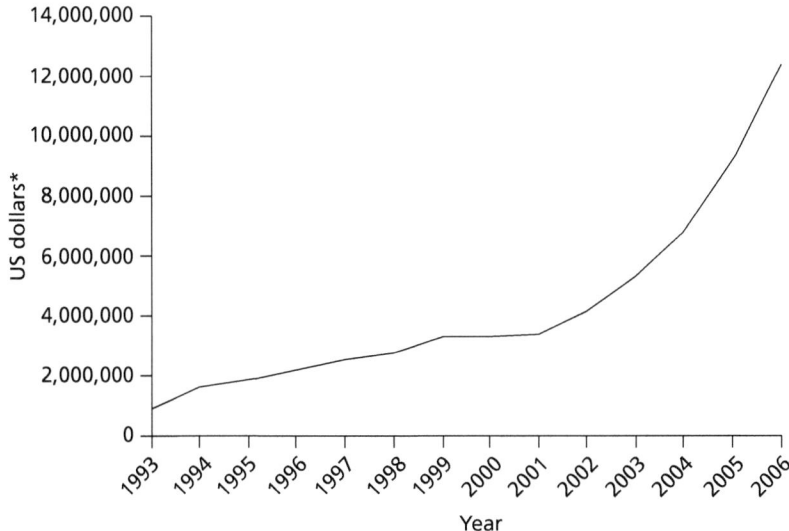

Figure 7.5 The growth in the wealth of the ILAE (in US $).
Source: data from International League Against Epilepsy (ILAE) Archive, http://www.ilae.org/visitors/ilae_archive/index.cfm, accessed 01 Oct. 2015.

The finances of the ILAE are an interesting study. Up until 1937, the turnover was very small, for example, £164 and 11 pence in 1937. The income raised was mainly from subscriptions from members and was spent mainly on producing the journal. In the early post-war years, finances improved, largely due to pharmaceutical company sponsorship of the congresses and advertising in the journal, and from the membership and conference fees coming from the enlarging number of chapters. By 1965, income was $6371 and this had risen by 1989 to $138 323. At that stage, the ILAE was still relatively small, with only 40 chapters and 1000 delegates at its international meetings. By then, income was derived largely from sponsorship, direct and indirect, from the manufacturers of carbamazepine and valproate which supported many conferences around the world. The phenomenal growth of the ILAE after 1990 has coincided with the rapid increase in the number of antiepileptic drugs, and much of ILAE income has derived from increasing sums of sponsorship from the burgeoning pharmaceutical industry of its congresses (both directly with satellites and stands and indirectly by sponsoring delegates) and journal. There are voices of protest suggesting that sponsorship from industry has reached levels which potentially compromise the integrity of the organisation, but as the activities have grown, so has the need maintain a healthy financial position. In recent times, more rigorous rules have been put in place to distance ILAE from the industry and a balance has been struck. At the time of writing, the central organisation of the ILAE has $17 million in its accounts, and the ILAE has therefore, in the past 20 years, been hugely successful financially. It has been the leading professional voice of epilepsy, but some have argued that with its focus on accruing finances, it is in danger of losing its way.

So what are the concrete achievements of the ILAE? Undoubtedly, the contributions made by its core activities, the journals and the congresses, to scientific and professional education have been indispensable. It, too, has exerted commendable policy influence, notably through the Global Campaign Against Epilepsy, which was launched in 1997 in partnership with the WHO and the ILAE's sister lay organisation the International Bureau for Epilepsy (IBE) (Figure 7.6), and more recently in 2011, the adoption of a written declaration on epilepsy in the European Parliament. The Global Campaign Against Epilepsy was its first major programme focusing on the problems of epilepsy in developing countries and it has put a stoplight on epilepsy where previously it had inhabited a world of shadows. In terms of professional policy, perhaps its most influential contribution has been its work on classification from 1964 to 1981 and that involved with pharmaceutical regulation in the 1970s. Nothing in recent times has matched these for importance or impact.

The ILAE has, since its inception, relied on a 'volunteer' culture. The officers, members of its taskforces and commissions, journal editors, and chapter

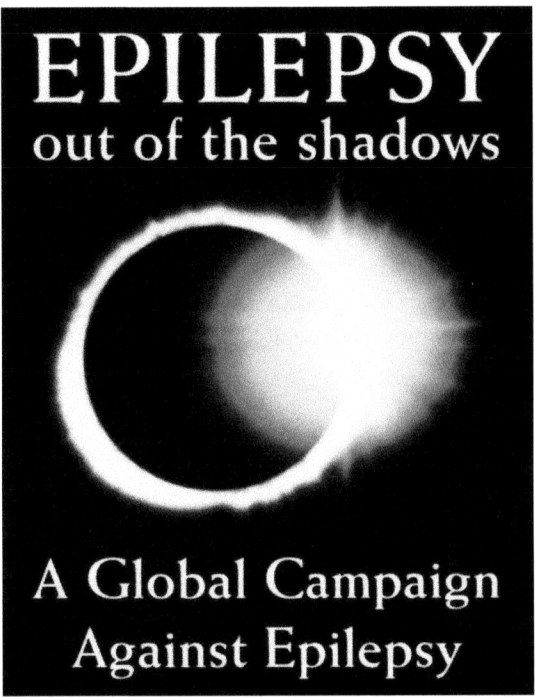

Figure 7.6 Logo of the ILAE/IBE/WHO Global Campaign Against Epilepsy entitled 'Out of the Shadows'.
Reproduced by kind permission of International League Against Epilepsy, Copyright © 2016 International League Against Epilepsy.

officials are all unpaid, and give their time freely, and this confers moral authority on the organisation. It was only in 1993 that the ILAE began to pay for secretarial support and in 2000 for professional administration and from 1999, too, ILAE has employed its own conference organising company. As the conferences have grown in size, greater professional assistance was clearly needed, and as the world becomes more globalised and more interconnected, there has also been a clear need for greater and more professional administration. However, the increasing and perhaps unavoidable bureaucratisation of the ILAE poses a threat, in our view, to the values of volunteerism which had characterised the League in its first hundred years. The unwelcome experience of meetings, often heavily concerned with money and politics, is a sign of this. It has, perhaps unfairly, been claimed by insiders that the focus has shifted too much from epilepsy towards endless debates about the processes of administration and finance. Constitutional changes are frequently made, and imperceptibly and without intending to, the organisation has turned inward, as has happened in other global organisations. One policy decision to maintain a large sum of money as an 'endowment' to ensure that the administrative costs can be met by the interest on this capital, is an example of the direction now taken. Some critics point out perhaps unjustly that in a medical world in which there are pressing problems in relation to providing education and in which the professionalism of clinicians is threatened, using keeping assets in this manner runs counter to its mission. ILAE also has, in recent times according to some critics directed a smaller percentage of its proceeds to its national chapters or regional commissions. This centralisation is to some these critics fear the consequence of its much enlarged administration, a classic example of the operation of Parkinson's law.

It could be argued that the greatest lost opportunity of the ILAE during its last 100 years was the failure to merge or to establish a closer and more equal relationship with its sister organisation, the IBE. The IBE was formed, as an international lay organisation in 1959, and within a decade the IBE and ILAE were working together. A merger was proposed in 1977. An umbrella organisation, *Epilepsy International*, was formed as a prelude to merger, but this collapsed in 1984 and was dismantled in 1987. The merger failed partly because the IBE could not adapt itself to the different perspective of the professional groups, and vice versa. The failed merger strained relationships initially but joint congresses have continued. The IBE is more financial straightened than the ILAE, but over the years requests for financial assistance from the ILAE have usually fallen on deaf ears. In the modern political climate, joint representations from professional and lay groups are a powerful lobby, and even if merger is not possible, it is to be hoped that the two organisations can continue to work closely together. The Global Campaign against Epilepsy is a remarkable example of what can be achieved by cooperation.

A bureaucratic issue which concerns the ILAE, and epilepsy more generally, and for which there is no easy solution, is that of the role of the pharmaceutical industry which has traditionally had an important role in oiling the wheels of postgraduate medical education. The industry sponsors conferences and meetings, at which they usually have advertising and stands, and sometimes run what is known as 'satellite symposia' which are separate sessions, added into the programme of the major conferences, and organised and financed by the companies. This is obviously open to potential abuse, but almost no congress would be able to survive financially without such industry support and ILAE for instance at its major conferences has charged over $100 000 for a stand and satellite symposium. The support of speakers and delegates to attend conferences has also become a political issue and source of adverse public comment. As an example from outside of the field of epilepsy, Merck in 2009 was forced to disclose that in a period of only 3 months it had paid out $3.7 million to US doctors to give lectures at conferences. As a consequence, pharmaceutical companies are now becoming ringed with stringent regulations about what is permissible. These regulations are designed to ensure that no unsubstantiated statements are made about any pharmaceutical product, and although most of this educational activity is entirely reputable, there is a perception that marketing rules continue to be abused. A report in 2011 showed that settlements of $15 billion in fines for fraudulent marketing had been paid by US drug companies in penalties in the previous 20 years. The main problem is off-label marketing and epilepsy drugs have been caught up in the centre of this.

As a result of the alleged abuse, increasingly strict conditions are currently being imposed on the pharmaceutical industry by national regulators, and an unintended consequence of this heavy-handed approach is that many educational events are now likely to go to the wall. Hospitals, universities, or individual doctors, it seems, are not prepared to fill the financial vacuum vacated by the industry.

The Bureaucracies of Drug Regulation and Guidelines: The Example of Epilepsy

The Food and Drug Administration (FDA) is the body responsible for implementing the US food and drug laws. It was formed initially as the US Department of Agriculture Bureau of Chemistry in 1906, and its main function was then to prevent misbranding and to ensure the strength, quality, and purity of drugs and of food. As mentioned in Chapter 4, regulations have over the years been greatly tightened in response to a series of scandals and disasters. Evidence of drug safety was first required in the 1930s, as a response to the scandal of the elixir of sulphanilamide. Then, in 1962, as a result of the thalidomide tragedy which was responsible for thousands of babies being born with abnormal limbs in Europe, but not in the United States,[5] the United States Congress passed the Kefauver–Harris Amendments, which for the first time required a standardised regimen of drug assessment (see Chapter 4). Those Amendments enshrined in law the absolute requirement that, before a drug company could put a new drug on the market, the manufacturer had to provide conclusive scientific evidence that the drug was 'safe', and for the first time, added the requirement that new drugs must also be proven to be 'effective'. They required that effectiveness be established by 'substantial evidence' which demonstrated that the drug will have the effects claimed in the drug's labelling. Substantial evidence was defined as consisting of 'adequate and well controlled investigations, including clinical investigations'. As described in

Chapter 3, the 1962 Amendments ushered in the modern era of drug evaluation and moved drug development and testing into the world of science. The FDA requirements became the 'gold standard' for the world.[6] The agency has grown in power and authority, and is a vast federal bureaucracy that regulates about a quarter of every dollar spent in the United States.

A description of the evolution of drug regulation, and especially in relation to the role of the FDA, is beyond the scope of this book, but this has been of central importance in defining the course of drug therapy in epilepsy. In Europe, individual countries had individual requirements for drug licensing until the formation of the European Medicines Agency (EMA) set up in 1995 to harmonise but not replace the individual national medicine regulatory bodies of EU members. The stated aim was to eliminate the protectionist tendencies of individual countries which had been prominent in the past and certainly still exists in many countries around the world (including the United States). The FDA and EMA regulations are similar in large part, although significant differences are found, for instance, in the monotherapy trial design in Europe for new-onset epilepsy where a non-inferiority design will suffice and not the need to demonstrate superiority as required by the FDA, and these issues are discussed further in Chapter 6.

The cost of carrying out all the investigations needed to bring a compound to market has been estimated to be in the region of $300 million and one concern frequently expressed is that the overbearing regulation may be a roadblock for innovation in the development of new drugs or devices. Do regulations inhibit the development of better drugs? There are arguments on both sides, and in the end the level of regulation is a societal decision based essentially on the level of risk that is deemed acceptable. What is clear though, is that the thousands of pages of regulations which now exist make seeing the wood for the trees very difficult. We will never know whether regulation has prevented new compounds which could have revolutionised antiepileptic therapy, but feel that this is quite possible.

For historical reasons, regulation has been focused on drug treatment, and the increasing number of 'devices' (stimulators and the like) have no such rigorous testing and the hurdles of proof for efficacy and safety are much lower. This is inconsistent and difficult to justify, and certainly our experience of some currently licensed stimulators is that they are only minimally effective, if at all. In passing, it is also of note that no surgical operation goes through any such rigorous evaluation and indeed surgeons are really at liberty to perform any operation as they wish, with only their professional bodies and the law courts providing any sanction over procedures carried out or standards of care.

The culture of 'guidelines' is another blooming bureaucracy that has arisen in many fields of medicine, including epilepsy. Obviously clinicians need advice, and clear and precise reasons for making their clinical choices, and authoritative guidelines can be very helpful, but the extraordinary proliferation of guidelines which now afflicts physicians trying to treat epilepsy is an avalanche, as described elsewhere, which 'risks burying the clinician in a white snow of double-talk and humbug' (19); this is no exaggeration. All sorts of agencies now produce 'guidelines' on the clinical management of epilepsy including governments, hospitals groups, professional bodies, and industry-sponsored groups and individuals. There are now even monthly guideline journals, some sponsored by the pharmaceutical industry.

Most guidelines purport to evaluate the medical qualities of a drug treatment. This is on top of the very detailed and rigorous procedures for drug licensing and the thousands of pages of regulations and armies of regulators involved in the drug licensing and pricing processes. Of course, the regulation of licensing has a narrow brief, and there are many issues relating to clinical practice issues which are not covered, but the irony of the current situation is that many of these clinical guidelines in epilepsy also tend to look narrowly at the clinical trial evidence in an attempt to appear 'scientific', and in the end adopt a perspective which is indistinguishable from that taken by the regulatory processes. This is a quite pointless duplication of effort.

Up until a few years ago, clinicians could exercise freedom to prescribe any drug licensed for the purpose, and exercise their independent judgement about its utility in any individual patient. They are now increasingly constrained by a second type of guideline produced at multiple levels of national or local organisations. In the United Kingdom, for instance, clinical guidelines are published by governmental or quasi-governmental agencies (e.g. National Institute for Health and Care Excellence (NICE) and Scottish Intercollegiate Guidelines Network (SIGN)) which exert great power and influence and often apply prescribing restrictions beyond those mandated in the licensing process. Professional bodies also produce guidelines, not least the local chapters of the ILAE for instance. Hospitals, too, have got in on the act, justified by the largely spurious claim that local issues can influence therapy, and the hospitals' formulary committees are some of the worse culprits in this guideline madness. The committees publish internal guidelines about which licensed drugs can be prescribed within the hospital group and to which category of patients, often without any special expertise, devoting a few minutes to any decision and yet claiming to be 'evidence based'. The resulting decisions are often alarmingly arbitrary.

On a darker note is the claim that guideline committees are themselves sometimes not independent. There are inevitable influences of personal prejudice and ego, but in addition, increasingly commonly, political pressures and commercial interference. Studies have repeatedly shown that commercially funded reviews are prone to bias in favour of the sponsor and the fact that guideline committees are frequently composed of individuals with potential conflicts of interest is concerning. The pharmaceutical industry recruits what it calls 'opinion leaders' and generously funds studies with often low scientific value, presumably primarily to influence opinion. The clinicians sitting on guideline committees have a responsibility to be objective, but in the face of personal reward, such objectivity is a fragile edifice.

There are also really important principles at stake in the current guideline culture, relating to clinical freedom and clinical responsibility. An individual patient consults a doctor on the understanding that the doctor will act in that individual's best interest, but a doctor surrounded by restrictive guidelines may not be able to deliver what he or she considers optimal advice. In the area of drug treatment, this seems to us inexcusable. Often the bureaucracies, in restricting treatment, claim the reason is financial, but in reality this is usually simply a matter of setting priorities, and physicians should fight their corner on behalf of a patient. Medicine is becoming increasingly thus bureaucratised, and in compromising the ability of a doctor to give best advice there is also an inevitable erosion of personal trust between doctor and patient.

There are legal implications too. Guidelines *are not* regulations but often are treated as such, and increasingly in litigation guidelines are used as evidence. The best clinical guidelines should provide a framework for the clinician who needs to weigh its advice and adapt it to the personal needs of an individual patient. This is a prerogative which must not be sacrificed at the altar of bureaucracy or overbearing regulation. A guideline should be just that, and not a rulebook.

Notes

1. For a comprehensive review of psychoanalytical theories, see Glover (5).
2. This whole issue is the topic of a number of excellent books (11–14).
3. For instance those of the International Committee of Medical Journal Editors, which states that the acquisition of funding, general supervision of the research group, or collection of data alone does not justify authorship.
4. The publications at the time of the ILAE centenary provide a detailed account of its evolution since 1909. These include Shorvon et al. (16,17).
5. Thalidomide's safety and effectiveness had been presented to the FDA by the pharmaceutical company Merrill. The drug had been developed by Gruenenthal in Aachen, Germany, and since 1957 had been widely sold in Europe and elsewhere as an excellent sedative. The fact that the drug was not licensed in the United States was due to the diligence of Dr Francis Kelsey (1914–2015), an FDA official who working with a chemist and a pharmacologist, found the evidence for Merrell's claims to be insufficient. She withheld approval despite great political pressure and was proved right when the reports of fetal damage began to surface.

6. More specifically, the requirement that a drug's effectiveness be demonstrated by 'adequate and well-controlled clinical investigations' has been interpreted by the FDA to mean a clinical study with: (i) clear objectives; (ii) adequate design to permit a valid comparison with a control group; (iii) adequate selection of study subjects; (iv) adequate measures to minimise bias; and (v) well-defined and reliable methods of assessing subjects' responses to treatment.

References

1. **Shorvon S.** The causes of epilepsy: changing concepts of etiology of epilepsy over the past 150 years. *Epilepsia* 2011; **52**(6):1033–1044.
2. **Friedlander WJ.** *The History of Modern Epilepsy: The Beginning, 1865-1914.* Westport CT: Greenwood Press; 2001.
3. **Jackson JH.** On the scientific and empirical investigation of epilepsies. *Med Press Circ* 1874; **18**:325–327, 347–352, 389–392, 409–412, 475–478, 497–499, 519–521.
4. **Nevins M.** *A Tale of Two 'Villages': Vineland and Skillman, NJ.* New York: iUniverse Inc; 2009.
5. **Glover E.** *Psycho-Analysis, A Handbook for Medical Practitioners and Students of Comparative Psychology*, 2nd ed. London: Staples Press; 1949:194–201.
6. **Dandy WE.** The practice of surgery. The brain. In: Lewis D (ed) *The Practice of Surgery*, Vol XII. Westport, CT: WF Prior; 1932.
7. **Gregoris N, Shorvon S.** What is the enduring value of research publications in clinical epilepsy? An assessment of papers published in 1981, 1991, and 2001. *Epilepsy Behav* 2013; **28**(3):522–529.
8. **Tallis R.** *Aping Mankind: Neuromania, Darwinitis and the Misrepresentation of Humanity.* Durham: Acumen; 2011.
9. **Rose S, Rose H.** *Genes, Cells and Brains: The Promethean Promises of the New Biology.* London: Verso; 2014.
10. **Ioannidis J.** Why most published research findings are false. *PloS Med* 2005; **2**(8): e124.
11. **Goldacre B.** *Bad Science.* London: Fourth Estate; 2009.
12. **Goldacre B.** *Bad Pharma.* New York: Faber and Faber; 2012.
13. **Healy D.** *Pharmageddon.* San Francisco, CA: University of California Press; 2013.
14. **Healy D.** *Mania: A Short History of Bipolar Disorder.* Baltimore, MD: Johns Hopkins University Press; 2010.
15. **Smith R.** *The Trouble with Medical Journals.* London: Royal Society of Medicine Press; 2006.
16. **Shorvon SD, Weiss G, Avanzini G,** et al. *International League Against Epilepsy 1909-2009: A Centenary History.* Oxford: Wiley Blackwell; 2009.
17. **Shorvon SD, Weiss G, Wolf P, Andermann F** (eds). To celebrate the centenary of Epilepsia and the ILAE: aspects of the history of epilepsy 1909–2009. *Epilepsia* 2009; **50**(Suppl 3):1–151.
18. **Shorvon SD.** Epilepsia—the journal of the International League Against Epilepsy In: Shorvon SD, Weiss G, Avanzini G, et al. *International League Against Epilepsy: A Centenary History.* Oxford: Wiley-Blackwell; 2009:163–206.
19. **Shorvon S.** We live in the age of the clinical guideline. *Epilepsia* 2006; **47**(7):1091–1093.

Chapter 8

Is the End of Epilepsy in Sight?

Although predictions are notoriously difficult, especially about the future, we felt it appropriate at the end of this book to speculate briefly how the future might bring the end of epilepsy. Of course the concepts are anecdotal and will probably not stand scrutiny in the future, but we here make a few suggestions anyway. Nor should we forget that it is always of interest to see what lessons for the future of drug treatment we can learn from the past.

All today is not doom. Current drug treatment of epilepsy is successful for many, if not for most people. The ultimate goal of treatment is, of course, the end of epilepsy and this is in reach for most patients. The best proxy for the end of epilepsy is complete and irreversible seizure remission without a need for further treatment, which at least marks the end of the biological condition if not all its societal and psychological consequences. The good news is that today the majority of people developing epilepsy will reach this goal after a few years of treatment. Complete seizure remission can be determined by following the course of epilepsy after cessation of drug treatment in patients who have become seizure free. Long-term studies have consistently shown that two out of three patients, when followed for one or more decades after they had their first seizure, will enter complete remission (usually defined as seizure remission without use of epilepsy drugs for at least 5 years) (1) (Figure 8.1). Unfortunately, though, not all patients can expect that their epilepsy will end when taking antiepileptic drugs, and it is for these patients that we seek improvements in the future.

Resolution of seizures is particularly important for families of children with epilepsy who often (but not always) have a good prognosis, and this explains why long-term outcome studies of childhood-onset epilepsy after stopping antiepileptic drugs have, deservedly, received great attention (2).[1] The end of epilepsy though is not easy to predict. During long-term follow-up, seizure remissions, often lasting several years, are interrupted by relapse in as many as one out of three patients. This is why any estimate of how many patients complete seizure remission is, to some extent, dependent on the length of the follow-up period. The most interesting question is of course who will be among the 60% with complete remission and how early one can predict the chance of complete remission. Uncomplicated epilepsy at the onset of disease, focal self-limited

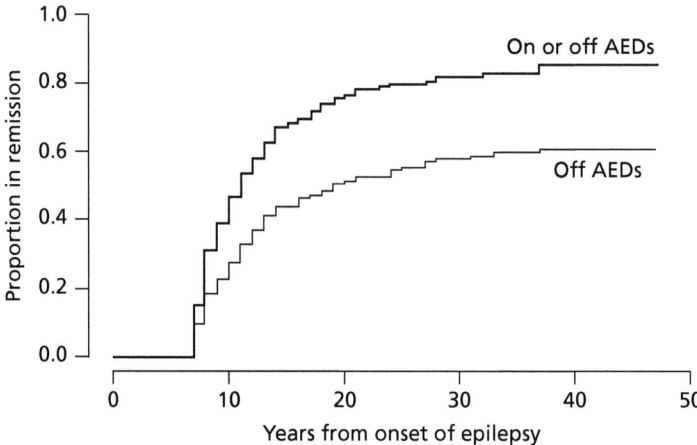

Figure 8.1 The end of epilepsy: about 60% of people with new-onset epilepsy enter a remission of at least 5 years after stopping antiepileptic drugs. Roughly 80% enter a remission of at least 5 years on or off antiepileptic drugs. Unfortunately, the 20% with persistent seizures and often additional brain disease that is responsible for the epilepsy have created the public image of an incurable condition.
Reproduced by kind permission of Maiju Saarinen and Mati Sillapää,
Copyright © 2016 Maiju Saarinen and Mati Sillapää.

epilepsy syndrome, uncharacterised epilepsy (that cannot easily be assigned to a specific epilepsy syndrome), and remission at 2 years after starting drug treatment point to a good chance of complete seizure remission (3).[2] Patients in remission who can be withdrawn from medications and remain seizure free for at least 5 years usually rapidly respond well to an antiepileptic drug. Most patients who have responded well to medications can stop taking antiepileptic drugs within 5–10 years. Reassuringly, long-term studies following antiepileptic drug withdrawal suggest that for the vast majority of people who become seizure free for several years after stopping antiepileptic drugs, the risk of having another seizure in the next 32 years is very small, in the range of 2% (1).

Understandably, not all patients in remission are willing to discontinue their medication. Compelling reasons for continuing medication can include anxiety of the patient or the physician that a relapse may occur after drug withdrawal, or concerns that a relapse may lead to loss of the job or the driver's licence. This is by no means rare: a study from Finland found out that as many as one out of six patients who are seizure free while taking medication are not keen to stop their epilepsy drugs (1).

The quest for a life without the burden and the risks of taking antiepileptic drugs every day is an aspiration for many. Drugs raise concerns about long-term adverse effects, especially teratogenic or cognitive or behavioural side effects, parents may wonder whether antiepileptic drugs do more harm than good for their child's developing brain, there are risks of adverse drug–drug interactions, there is a cost of monitoring and follow-up care, and taking drugs reinforces the sense of being sick. In children, too, there is a concern that cumulative, even minor, effects of antiepileptic drugs may permanently affect their educational progress and eventual intellectual functioning and this possibility of course is very difficult to prove or disprove. After years of antiepileptic drug use, its true influence on cognitive functioning is often only fully appreciated once the particular drug is discontinued. Although stopping antiepileptic drugs is associated with improvement on some cognition scales, although not IQ, perhaps surprisingly, it has been found that the quality of life does not regularly improve when antiepileptic drugs are stopped.

The taking of drugs is an issue, as always, of risk versus benefit, and although there are some benefits to discontinuation, this has to be balanced against the risk of seizure recurrence (4).[3] A benchmark study from Liverpool, United Kingdom, authoritatively determined that the risk of seizure recurrence after discontinuing antiepileptic drugs was twice as high over the next 2 years compared with staying on medication (5). Relapses mostly occurred in the first year of withdrawal and adults are generally more at risk than children. The societal effects of seizure relapse are also generally somewhat greater in adults than in children. A seizure relapse in public or at the workplace can be embarrassing and stigmatising, and may destroy careers. A particular threat is losing the driver's licence. Furthermore, one perhaps unexpected twist is the observation that restarting antiepileptic drugs after recurrence does not always guarantee immediate and complete remission in as many as one out of five adults. Recurrence on drug withdrawal also carries the risk of accidents, which fortunately are rare, and has been implicated as a cause of SUDEP. The decision about whether to withdraw medication is therefore a difficult one, and striking a balance between the pros and cons, and considering factors which are difficult to compare will in the end depend a great deal on the patient's attitude to risk.

In passing it should be noted that some patients with apparent epilepsy, unresponsive to treatment, are in fact misdiagnosed and a common error is the over-interpretation of the EEG in someone who has had a blackout of some sort. The skill of the treating physician in choosing medication and acting when medication is not working are also important. In general, though, patients who do not have good control with medications after the first year are more likely to have difficulty with epilepsy treatment for many years than those who enter quick remission. Other factors associated with difficult-to-control epilepsy include having several types of seizures, an abnormal EEG or MRI, and abnormal neurological exam. For those with drug refractory epilepsy, brain surgery can be the only realistic option to enter complete remission off antiepileptic drugs, and this is itself often a risky option with no guarantee of success.

New Thinking and New Strategies for Drug Development

As outlined in earlier chapters, there are limitations of current drug treatments which weigh heavily on patients with chronic or severe epilepsy and we need new strategies of drug development. The bottom line is that a revolution in discovery and development is needed. Drug development is alive and well, as seen by the number of potential antiepileptic drugs in clinical trials (Table 8.1)

Future antiepileptic drugs, however, are expected to show added clinical value over what we have now, as now requested by many regulatory agencies (except curiously in the United States). This raises the bar for the pharmaceutical industry, but is in our opinion a welcome test.

Our understanding of the mechanisms mediating the development of epilepsy and the causes of drug resistance has grown substantially over the past decade providing opportunities for the discovery and preclinical development of more efficacious antiseizure, antiepileptogenic, and disease-modifying drugs for prevention. The fashionable mantra of the moment is the belief that the best approach for minimising risk in clinical development is so-called target-related development (6) (Figure 8.2) in which a drug is selected that

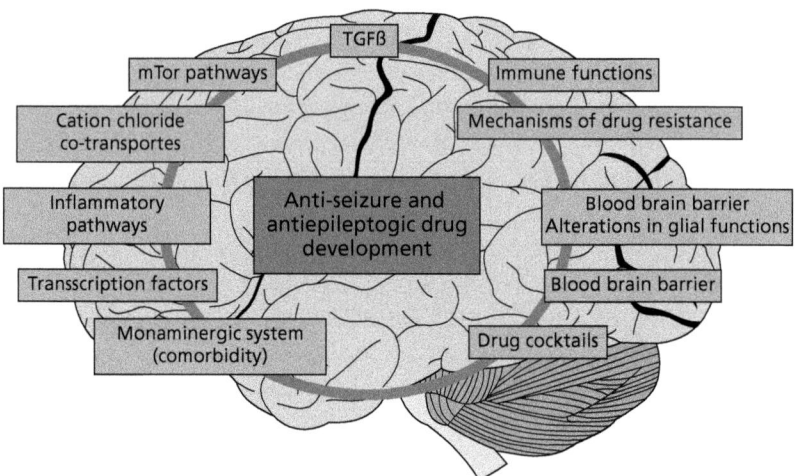

Figure 8.2 Potential future therapies for seizures and epilepsies. Things are getting more complicated than in the past when antiepileptic drugs were mostly small molecules. Examples of novel targets that are particularly interesting for development of antiseizure and anti-epileptogenic drugs are shown.
Adapted with permission from Löscher W, Klitgaard H, Twyman RE, and Schmidt D. New avenues for anti-epileptic drug discovery and development. *Nature Reviews Drug Discovery*, Volume 12, Issue 10, pp. 757–76, Copyright © 2013 Macmillan Publishers Ltd.

has a well-documented mechanism of action clearly associated with a positive therapeutic effect in epilepsy.

Repurposing existing drugs which were developed for other indications or using alternative delivery methods or formulations, is another current approach. A variety of recently discovered pathways and potential drug targets show considerable promise in this regard (6) (Figure 8.3).

Most epilepsies though are not likely to result from alterations in a single target; rather, they will arise from complex system changes. Thus, single-target treatments that focus exclusively on a single protein or individual biochemical pathway might well be less effective than multiple-target treatments that act on different proteins or pathways involved in the network. The latter approach—multitarget treatment—has been recently termed 'network pharmacology' or 'pleotherapy'. The approach of network pharmacology is to develop combinations of existing drugs or novel drugs that modulate several mechanisms and regulate activity at different points within a biological network. Systems biology-based approaches of network pharmacology have recently been proposed for the development of both antiepileptic and antiepileptogenic treatments (1).

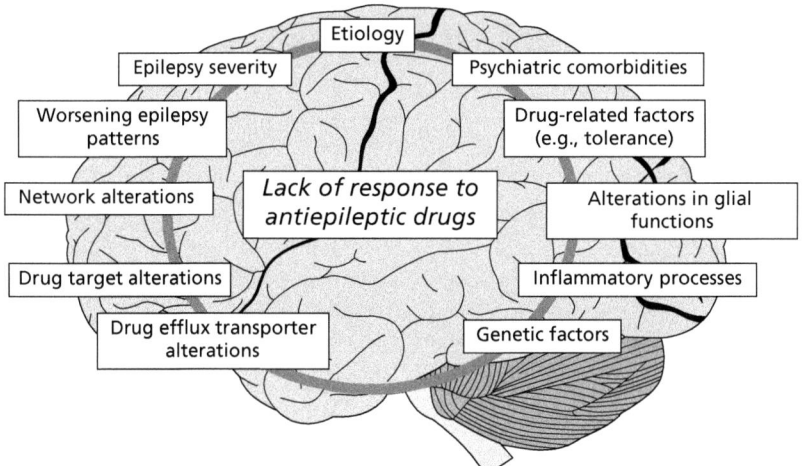

Figure 8.3 Potential future therapies for drug-resistant epilepsy What we are up against when developing new treatment(s) of prior drug-resistant epilepsy is illustrated in this figure. Rather diverse factors may contribute to make an antiepileptic drug work and, more importantly, may prevent response in drug-resistant epilepsy. Not surprisingly we are still struggling to find a single treatment for drug resistance.
Adapted with permission from Löscher W, Klitgaard H, Twyman RE, and Schmidt D. New avenues for anti-epileptic drug discovery and development. *Nature Reviews Drug Discovery*, Volume 12, Issue 10, pp. 757–76, Copyright © 2013 Macmillan Publishers Ltd.

Table 8.1 Potential antiepileptic drugs in clinical trials as discussed at the Eilat Congresses 1994–2014

Eilat II, 1994	Eilat III, 1996	Eilat IV, 1998	Eilat V, 2000	Eilat VI, 2002	Eilat VII, 2004
Dezinamide	Dezinamide	534U87	AWD 131–138	Carabersat (SB- 204269)	Atipamezole
Levetiracetam (UCB L059)	Levetiracetam (UCB L059)	ADCI	DP-VPA (DP16)	Conantokin-G (CGX-1007)	BIA 2-093
Losigamone	Ralitoline	AWD 131–138	Harkeroside (SPM 927)	Pregabalin	Brivaracetam (UCB 34714)
Remacemide hydrochloride	Remacemide	DP16 (DP-VPA)	LY 300164	Retigabine	Fluorofelbamate
Rufinamide (CGP 33101)	Retigabine (D-23129)	Ganaxolone (CCD 1042)	NPS 1776	Safinamide	NPS 1776
Stiripentol	Rufinamide (CGP 33101)	Levetiracetam (UCB LO59)	NW-1015	SPD421 (DP-VPA)	Pregabalin
Tiagabine	Tiagabine	Losigamone	Pregabalin (CI-1008)	SPM 927	Retigabine
Topiramate	TV 1901	Pregabalin (CI-1008; isobutyl GABA)	Remacemide	Talampanel	RWJ-333369
		Remacemide hydrochloride	Retigabine (D-23129)	Valrocemide (TV 1901)	Safinamide
		Retigabine (D-29129)	Rufinamide		SPM 927
		Rufinamide (CGP 33101)	Valrocemide (TV 1901)		Stiripentol
		Soretolide (D2916)			Talampanel
		TV 190112			Valrocemide

Reproduced with permission Shorvon SD. Historical Introduction. In: Shorvon S, Perucca E, Engel J, *The Treatment of Epilepsy*, 4th edition. Oxford: Wiley-Blackwell, Copyright © 2015 John Wiley and Sons, Ltd.

Eilat VIII, 2006	Eilat IX, 2008	Eilat X, 2010	Eilat XI, 2012	Eilat XII, 2014
Brivaracetam (UCB 34714)	2-Deoxy-o-glucose	2-Deoxy-o-glucose	2-Deoxy-o-glucose	2-Deoxy-o-glucose
Eslicarbazepine acetate (BIA 2-093)	Brivaracetam (UCB 34714)	Brivaracetam	Brivaracetam	Adenosine-releasing silk
Fluorofebamate	Carisbamate (RWJ-333369)	Carisbamate	Ganaxolone	Allopregnanolone
Ganaxolone	Eslicarbazepine acetate (BIA 2-093)	Ganaxolone	ICA-105665	AMP-X-0079
Huperzine A	Fluorofebamate	Huperzine A	Imepitoin	BGG492
JZP-4	Ganaxolone	ICA-105665	NAX-810-2	Brivaracetam
Lacosamide	Huperzine A	NAX-5055	Perampanel	Bumetamide
NS1209	JZP-4	Perampanel	Propylisopropyl acetamide (PID)	Butylpropylacetamide (SPD
Propylisopropyl acetamide (PID)	Lacosamide (SPM 927)	Propylisopropyl acetamide (PID)	Tonabersat	Cannabidiol
Retigabine	NAX 5055	Retigabine	Valnoctamide (VCD)	Cannbidivarin (GWP 420006)
Rufinamide	Propylisopropyl acetamide (PID)	T2007 (sodium 5,5-diphenylbarbiturate)	VK-765	Everolimus
RWJ-333369	Retigabine	Valnoctamide (VCD)	YKP3089	Ganaxolone
Seletracetam (UCB 44212)	T2000	YKP3089		Huperzine A
Stiripentol	Tonabersat			Imepitoin
Talampanel	Valnoctamide			Micocycline
Valrocemide	Valrocemide			NAX-810-2
	YKP3089			Pitolisant (Tiprolisant)
				Propofol hemisuccinate
				Propylisopropyl acetamide (PID)
				PRX 0023 (Naluzotan)
				SAGE-217
				Valnoctamide (VCD)
				VLB-01
				YKP3089

Network pharmacology could also tackle another challenge of drug development—that many drugs work on only a subset of patients. By performing network analysis of individual patients, inter-individual variations of disease mechanisms might be identified, enabling clinical trials to be carried out in groups of patients who share the same underlying molecular condition. For example, by using biomarkers, patients with a specific mechanism of resistance can be identified and treated with a drug targeting this mechanism. Indeed, biomarkers for a specific mechanism of drug resistance would be required before the clinical trial investigator could effectively recruit a sufficiently large enough sample size. How realistic this hope is, long expressed and yet still undelivered, is a moot point.

Some drug combinations have demonstrated substantial synergy and are strikingly more effective in models of seizure and epilepsy than each compound alone. This approach does present both opportunities and complications for intellectual property rights and commercialisation. The benefits of repurposing existing drugs include diminished development time and costs. Interest in the pharmaceutical industry does appear to exist and large pharmaceutical companies, biotech companies, and academic laboratories are forming consortia for network pharmacology.

The development of specific therapies for individual types of seizures that have been neglected up to now, for instance specific therapies for tonic–clonic seizures, would present a breakthrough as uncontrolled tonic–clonic seizures are a major risk factor for SUDEP. In addition, we need new and better drugs for rare but life-threatening epilepsy syndromes such as Lennox–Gastaut syndrome (6). The discovery that vigabatrin has unique action in West syndrome, a rare but often devastating epilepsy of infancy, and stiripentol for Dravet syndrome are examples of such specificity, but interestingly each indication was found by chance, long after the drugs had been tested in more common types of seizures.

The adverse effects of antiepileptic drugs are another big challenge. Currently, at least 50% of patients complain of side effects, and all antiepileptic drugs manifest these to varying degrees. Furthermore, the classical preclinical screening models in mice and rats, such as the MES and PTZ tests, have consistently selected drugs which have significant neurological side effects, apparently as a result of the type of models used. One technical issue that makes it difficult to assess the safety and tolerability of new drugs is that current trial designs are usually statistically powered to detect treatment effects on seizures but do not include enough patients to assess uncommon side effects seen in a few per cent of patients. As a consequence, the risk of serious adverse events may only be discovered at a late stage in the adoption of new antiepileptic drugs, such as idiosyncratic events or toxic effects that are difficult to identify and predict from preclinical development programmes. Felbamate, vigabatrin, and, most recently, retigabine are examples among new antiepileptic drugs that turned out to have substantial side effects that were not discovered in the clinical trials which usually include no more than 3000 patients. There is emerging evidence that individual genetic factors predispose to having higher rates of side effects (7)[4] and knowledge of these has the promise of developing personalising medicines—a much hyped possibility for many years, but currently very little progress has been made.

Why is it so difficult to develop a better drug for epilepsy? One reason is that taking a drug from the laboratory and preclinical testing arena into first-in-human studies and clinical trials represents the largest, most costly gamble in the drug discovery pipeline. During this phase of development, patient safety takes centre stage and acquires quantifiable parameters, dosing may require some guesswork and trial-and-error, unexpected toxicities and off-target effects may arise, and the first real sense of how a compound will be processed, metabolised, made available to tissues and cells, and affect normal physiology and disease becomes evident. About one-third of experimental drugs never make it past the first phase I of trials in healthy volunteers and only about 13% of those that enter clinical testing receive market approval. Nearly two-thirds of drugs that make it past early clinical trials in patients with epilepsy (phase II trials) fail in late-stage phase III studies, following a substantial investment of time, money, and resources.

Another aspect of new thinking about drug treatment is in fact old thinking—and that is the use of alternative or complementary medicine. There is a long history of this in epilepsy, and despite repeated dismissal by orthodox practitioners, usually on the basis that there is 'no evidence' of effectiveness, it remains popular among patients usually for reasons such as disillusionment with conventional therapy due to lack of effect or side effects, or often a deep suspicion about the potential adverse effects, as yet unrecognised, caused by powerful pharmaceuticals, a concern which has some historical justification in the case, for instance, of drugs such as thalidomide or paracetamol. Felbamate is an example in the field of epilepsy. Felbamate was discovered to cause life-threatening liver and blood disease only after thousands of patients received it after it entered the market. Many also have an intuitive dislike of the idea of being dependent for life on medication and prefer the concept of working with 'nature' or nature bodily rhythms. A patient recently said that she would prefer rain forest drugs instead of chemicals, somewhat disingenuously of course given that we, and every animal and plant, are anyway biochemicals. In fact, many patients take, in addition to their antiepileptic drugs, pills and concoctions bought from health-food stores or practitioners of traditional medicines. The list of such unorthodox treatments is long and ranges from Ayurveda pills causing harm either because of toxic components such as lead or the use of homeopathic pills, with substances in ridiculously low concentrations, or herbal medicines used for centuries with no evidence of effectiveness, or miscellaneous vitamins, chemicals, animal or plant toxins, aromatherapy, acupuncture, or psychological and physical treatments. In 2005, a survey of patients in the United Kingdom (8) found that 34% of patients with epilepsy had used a complementary medicine at some point in time, and most had not informed their doctor, and in a survey in Germany (9) among parents of children with epilepsy, 37% had used alternative therapies in the previous year of which homeopathy, osteopathy, and kinesiology were the most common. It is worth remembering, too, that few of these materials have had rigorous testing of safety or efficacy, yet are preferred above allopathic medicine despite the fact that this is highly regulated. Interestingly, patients who are very suspicious about side effects of antiepileptic drugs are much less worried about the risks of such unproven medication, and this is despite the lack of the sort of regulatory oversight that applies to orthodox medicines. In the age of the Internet, too, there are wild and unsubstantiated claims available for all to see for many treatments, and the fact that these are taken in addition to, or in place of, conventional medicines is to an extent an indictment of modern medicine.

Why are patients willingly exposing themselves to such potentially harmful substances? Failure of orthodox medical treatment and the desire for better treatment elsewhere is an understandable motivation. Other reasons are a desire to take control, a desire to escape the restrictions of a lifestyle imposed by an overbearing medical system, and the tyranny of doctors, documentation, doctors' notes, and hospital notes and letters. Many also feel a lack of respect and dignity when exposed to short office visits lasting a few minutes after waiting often for hours. Some would rather pay and stay under the radar of official documentation. Taken together, the fact that untried, expensive, and potentially dangerous alternative or complementary therapies are sought is a litmus test for the failure of our current medical system. Alternative methods of therapy rely a great deal on the perceived benefits of a 'holistic' approach, and such approaches were strongly advocated by epilepsy doctors in the pre-pharmaceutical age. In our so-called evidence-based medicine, these aspects are neglected by many practitioners and should be re-examined. Have we thrown the baby out with the bathwater? Probably so. Ironically, several of the largest pharmaceutical companies are involved in active research into the potential of many traditional herbal therapies.

A related point concerns the potential benefit of placebo. Traditionally placebos have been used in epilepsy as a methodological tool in clinical trials to identify ineffective and harmful treatments (see Chapter 6). Curiously, many patients do quite well on placebos themselves, and research into placebo effects can help explain mechanistically how clinicians can be therapeutic agents in the ways they relate to their patients in connection with, and separate from, providing biologically active interventions. Of course, placebo effects are modest as compared with the impressive results achieved by life-saving surgery and powerful, well-targeted medications (10), but although placebo effects are often dismissed as the negligible effects of an 'inert substance', this underestimates their scope, the complexity, and the clinical significance. In a broad sense, placebo effects are attributable to a patient's participation in the therapeutic encounter, with its rituals, symbols, identifiable health-care paraphernalia and settings, emotional and cognitive engagement with clinicians, empathic and intimate witnessing, and the laying on of hands (7). Placebo effects have also been shown to rely on complex neurobiological mechanisms involving neurotransmitters and activation of specific, quantifiable, and relevant areas of the brain. Recent clinical research into placebo effects has provided compelling evidence that these effects are genuine biopsychosocial phenomena that represent more than simply spontaneous remission, normal symptom fluctuations, and regression to the mean (4).

Placebos may provide relief, yet they rarely cure. Although research has revealed objective neurobiological pathways and correlates of placebo responses, the evidence to date suggests that the therapeutic benefits associated with placebo effects do not alter the pathophysiology of diseases beyond their symptomatic manifestations; they primarily address subjective and self-appraised symptoms (11). To be fair, that is exactly what our current antiepileptic drugs are doing. Our current antiepileptic drugs, though welcome, have not been convincingly shown to do anything but bring symptomatic relief through suppression of seizures.

Should we consider non-traditional study designs in epilepsy? The recently introduced 21st Century Cures Act in the United States instructs the FDA to consider non-traditional study designs and methods of data analysis to further speed approvals (12). Adaptive trial designs and the use of Bayesian methods hold promise in some kinds of evaluations, particularly in oncology. However, more problematic proposals include encouraging the use of 'shorter or smaller clinical trials' for devices and the request that the FDA develop criteria for relying on 'evidence from clinical experience', including 'observational studies, registries, and therapeutic use' instead of randomised controlled trials for approving new uses for existing drugs. Such data can provide important information about drug utilisation and safety once a medication is in use. However, these approaches are not as rigorous or valid as randomised trials in assessing efficacy.

Recently an oncology drug (Keytruda) was given accelerated approval by the FDA, allowing it to reach the market without the three typical phases of clinical trials needed to show a drug can prolong lives. Keytruda was approved based on what was essentially an extra-large phase I trial involving 173 participants who all received the drug, with no control group. Tumours shrank in about 24% of patients, the FDA said, with the effect lasting at least 1.4–8.5 months and continuing beyond this period in most patients. Even the very preliminary results on a handful of patients, 20 or so, indicated a high degree of activity. The pharmaceutical company will now have to conduct two controlled clinical trials to verify that the drug can prolong lives and delay the progression of disease (14). Could a similar approach be taken in epilepsy?

Consider this idea for yourself. Should we pay only when a costly drug works? If drug treatment for epilepsy becomes more costly, as it undoubtedly will, one interesting idea to limit costs would be to pay only when it works. Unless a previously defined benefit is shown, treatment costs are refunded by the drug company. Examples exist outside of epilepsy. In Germany, insurance companies have agreements for patients with severe allergic asthma. If their treatment with a costly drug does not work, the treatment costs are refunded by the pharmaceutical company.

Finally and in summary, what shall we do to have better drugs for epilepsy in the future? A group of clinical and experimental scientists from academia and industry proposed a roadmap for the discovery and development of medications for drug-resistant epilepsy and for epilepsy prevention or disease modification (6). According to this proposal, following the identification of novel targets or compounds, extensive pharmacological and/or genetic validation would be required before making the decision to initiate further drug discovery efforts. These efforts would aim to identify a preclinical candidate (or candidates) that can subsequently be validated in comparative, preclinical proof-of-concept studies. Translation to phase I studies would involve the use of PET ligands and other biomarkers to assess target engagement and to conduct early, decisive, but less costly proof-of-concept 'light' studies, which reveal whether a biological consequence of target engagement can be detected by imaging, EEG, or other biomarkers. This would be followed by a comparative, add-on phase II study in patients, in which the magnitude of the efficacy signal determines the potential of pursuing confirmatory add-on phase III studies at a later stage, which would involve making a direct comparison between the drug and the standard of care, if any (6).

A major incentive for the industry to adopt this strategy and to execute it successfully will be the availability of valid targets amenable to drug therapy, interpretable and target-population-relevant pre-clinical proof-of-concept studies, disease and target-related biomarkers, diagnostic methodology for the identification of the specific patient populations, and innovative clinical trial designs. Fortunately, various initiatives from major public and private funding bodies in the United States and Europe have recently stimulated a focus on further identification of these concepts, and this has led to new concerted efforts between academia and industry. This holds potential for the revitalisation of antiepileptic drug discovery and development, bringing us closer to the ultimate goal of curing epilepsy.

Antiepileptogenesis and Prevention

The ability of a drug to prevent epilepsy, not just block seizures which are the main symptoms of epilepsy, is called antiepileptogenesis (1), and the development of drugs for this purpose is perhaps the most challenging goal for future pharmaceutical research (13).[5] This is no trivial task as investigators and pharmaceutical companies have learned in the last 40 years. How could a drug possibly be demonstrated to prevent epilepsy? The only way to do this in a practical setting is to identify patients at high risk of getting epilepsy in the future, and to use medication possibly even prior to the first seizure in such patients. As many as 40% of all patients develop epilepsy after severe traumatic brain injury, ischaemic stroke, intracerebral haemorrhage, or encephalitis. Although epileptogenesis can start immediately at the time of an acute injury (14), often there is a delay. More than 130 years ago, Gowers (1881; see Appendix) first recognised that there is an enigmatic seizure-free interval, called the latent period, lasting months to years, between brain insult and the onset of epilepsy. The interval between injury and the first seizure is the first 'window of opportunity' for drugs to stop epileptogenesis (14).[6] A widely accepted hypothesis holds that during this seizure-free latent period, which characterises many cases of symptomatic epilepsy, there is a cascade of poorly understood changes that transform the healthy brain into one that generates spontaneous recurrent seizures. Numerous possible mechanisms underlying this process of epileptogenesis have been suggested, but no consensus has emerged about which of the observed changes is causal, and how they interact (14). Sadly, no trial has to date been successful in preventing acquired epilepsy. The methodological problems are formidable.

One promising method for improving the feasibility of antiepileptogenic prevention trials is to identify 'biomarkers' of epilepsy, and trial the drug in patients in whom these biomarkers are present. Biomarkers could in theory be clinical factors, laboratory results, EEG or MRI features. EEG alterations such as pre-ictal spikes or high-frequency oscillations (known as ripples), are examples of potentially useful biomarkers. Bioinformatics and network-based systems biology approaches are already used in neurotrauma and Alzheimer's disease research, and could possibly be applied to identify the most predictive combination of biomarkers for the various types of epilepsy.

A promising area for future antiepileptogenic drug trials is to test them in patients with drug-resistant epilepsy with the aim to limit or to abolish the disease process that is causing the drug-resistant epilepsy. This treatment is called disease modification. Specific drugs are currently being developed that may possibly need only be given for weeks or months to exert their long-lasting effect. Disease-changing treatment can be assessed prospectively in a double-blind design in patients with epilepsy who are seizure free after surgery and plan to discontinue antiepileptic drug treatment (5). A disease-changing treatment would prevent relapse of seizures which are seen on average in one out of three patients when antiepileptic drugs are withdrawn in patients with sustained seizure freedom on antiepileptic drugs (1). Finally, adding a disease-modifying agent could further improve the prognosis of new-onset epilepsy. These are all scenarios for future efforts to bring the end of epilepsy to more patients than we can do today.

The Real End of Epilepsy

Temkin chose the title 'The end of falling sickness?' as the title of the last section of his famous book, not because he thought it likely that epilepsy as a medical condition would disappear, on the contrary, he noted that its biological nature as far as we can tell has not changed much in recorded history, but because he hoped that it might cease being a 'paradigm of the suffering of both body and soul in disease'. Obviously the complete control of seizures is a most important element in this, but not the only one. If medicinal methods for completely suppressing seizures do not prove possible, and if methods for preventing epilepsy are not developed, it was his hope, and is ours, that the fact of having epileptic seizures can in the future not carry the baggage of history, social oppression, and stigma that has so afflicted patients in the past and now.

Epilepsy is, as pointed out throughout this book, however, more than just having seizures. Seizures are sometimes accompanied by physical and biological co-morbidities such as depression and psychological disturbances, issues of self-esteem and confidence, neurological signs and intellectual impairments, and an association with other non-neurological conditions which might be related to underlying constitutional derangements or epilepsy therapy. Those extra factors which are biological in nature will hopefully be susceptible to scientific management and cure, and for this we rely on scientific research and innovation. Science has advanced enormously in many areas and we are confident that many of such co-morbidities of epilepsy will be quickly understood. The non-biological aspects though, the societal aspects of epilepsy which have been so heavy a burden for patients to bear in the past, as briefly illustrated in Chapter 2, can be alleviated only with changes in social attitude and mores. This is in the hands of all citizens and is a responsibility for society, not a duty of science or medicine narrowly defined. In our view, there has been much to celebrate in recent decades and the plight of the person with epilepsy has been greatly improved, but still much needs to be done. The creation of a society that does not denigrate disability or shun the vulnerable or the afflicted, that treats individuals as worthy and celebrates their achievements and their very existence, is in the gift of all of us. This does not require laboratory facilities, markets, industry, or research funding. It is an attitude change; deconstructing the condition so that it no longer is a paradigm of the suffering of the soul, as much as of the body, would indeed mark the true end of epilepsy.

Notes

1. The National General Practice Study of Epilepsy and other studies for example in Finland have shown that:

    (i) epilepsy has an often good prognosis with 65–85% of cases eventually entering long-term remission, and an even higher proportion of cases entering a short-term remission; (ii) the likelihood of long-term remission of seizures is much better in newly diagnosed cases than in patients with chronic epilepsy; (iii) the early response to treatment is a good guide to longer term prognosis (although not inevitably so, as in a minority of cases seizure remission can develop after prolonged activity); (iv) the longer is the remission (and follow-up), the less likely is subsequent recurrence; (v) the longer an epilepsy is active, the poorer is the longer-term outlook; (vi) that delaying treatment, even for many years, does not worsen long-term prognosis; (vii) the 'continuous' and 'burst' patterns are more common than the 'intermittent' seizure pattern; (viii) epilepsy has a mortality that is highest in the early years after diagnosis, and in the early years is largely due to the underlying cause, however, higher mortality rates than expected are observed throughout the course of an epilepsy; (ix) the prognosis of febrile seizures is generally good, with ~6–7% developing later epilepsy; and (x) clinical factors associated with outcome have been well studied, and those consistently found to predict a worse outcome include: the presence of neurodeficit, high frequency of seizures before therapy (seizure density), poor response to initial therapy, some epilepsy syndromes (2).

2. Four independent factors were found to be associated with long-term epilepsy cure compared with having seizures while on antiepileptic drugs: seizure frequency less than

in medically treated patients, the risk of recurrence after antiepileptic drug withdrawal is increased until 2 years after withdrawal, although long-term seizure outcomes seem to be unaffected by drug policies. Most relapses occur during the first year after withdrawal. Several predictors of relapse have been identified. The risk of developing uncontrollable epilepsy following withdrawal is less than one in five. There is no proof that antiepileptic drug withdrawal itself negatively affects long-term seizure outcomes in patients who became seizure free under antiepileptic drug treatment or after epilepsy surgery. Antiepileptic drug discontinuation unveils the natural history of the epilepsy in medically treated patients, and the completeness of resection of the epileptogenic network in patients who underwent epilepsy surgery. Early during the first 12 months of antiepileptic drug treatment, pretreatment seizure frequency less than weekly, higher IQ (>70), and no symptomatic aetiology of epilepsy. Patients with seizure frequency of less than once a week during early treatment and no evidence for symptomatic aetiology had a ninefold chance of being cured since the onset of the first adequate antiepileptic therapy until the end of follow-up compared with patients who a symptomatic aetiology had at least weekly seizures while on antiepileptic drugs. In conclusion, IQ, aetiology, and seizure frequencies both in the first year of antiepileptic drug treatment and prior to medication appear to be clinical predictors of cure in childhood-onset epilepsy (3).

3. In medically treated patients, the risk of recurrence after antiepileptic drug withdrawal is increased until 2 years after withdrawal, although long-term seizure outcomes seem to be unaffected by drug policies. Most relapses occur during the first year after withdrawal. Several predictors of relapse have been identified. The risk of developing uncontrollable epilepsy following withdrawal is less than one in five. There is no proof that antiepileptic drug withdrawal itself negatively affects long-term seizure outcomes in patients who became seizure-free under antiepileptic drug treatment or after epilepsy surgery. Antiepileptic drug discontinuation unveils the natural history of the epilepsy in medically treated patients, and the completeness of resection of the epileptogenic network in patients who underwent epilepsy surgery (4).

4. Pharmacogenetic alterations might potentially affect efficacy, tolerability. Examples that have been studied include variation in genes encoding drug target (SCN1A), drug transport (ABCB1), drug metabolising (CYP2C9, CYP2C19), and human leucocyte antigen (HLA) proteins. Although the current studies associating particular genes and their variants with seizure control or adverse events have inherent weaknesses and have not provided unifying conclusions, several results, for example, that Asian patients with a particular HLA allele, HLA-B*1502, are at a higher risk for Stevens–Johnson syndrome when using carbamazepine, are helpful to increase our knowledge of how genetic variation affects the treatment of epilepsy. Although genetic testing raises ethical and social issues, a better understanding of the genetic influences on epilepsy outcome may be a key to developing the much needed new therapeutic strategies for individuals with epilepsy (7).

5. A wide variety of experimental studies and clinical trials using chronic antiseizure drug therapy during the extended post-injury period have had minimal success. The disappointing results of these studies may be due to several factors including the possibility that antiseizure drugs, despite the fact they suppress seizure activity, do not interfere in any substantial way with the 'epileptogenic' process of focal epilepsies. Although the reasons for the failure are not entirely clear, it may be that the antiseizure drugs may have

been tested at the wrong doses, for the wrong duration, or at the wrong time after brain injury. Surprisingly, the anti-absence drug ethosuximide has also been shown to be antiepileptogenic in several experimental models of absence epilepsy. In addition, clinical trials aimed at preventing focal post-injury epilepsy have suffered from poor enrolment and other issues related to the co-morbidity of severe epilepsies that follow overt brain injury. Testing specific anti-inflammatory and immunological antiepileptogenic agents to prevent focal epilepsies, as well as prevention trials for genetic epilepsies, possibly with anti-absence drugs, may be a way to resolve the dilemma. Although more evidence is needed, there is hope on the horizon for antiepileptogenic therapy that works (13).

6. This review, based on recent data from both animal models and patients with different types of brain injury, proposes that epileptogenesis and often subclinical epilepsy can start immediately after brain injury without any appreciable latent period. Even though the latent period has traditionally been the cornerstone concept representing epileptogenesis, we suggest that the evidence for the existence of a latent period is spotty both for animal models and human epilepsy. Knowing whether a latent period exists or not is important for our understanding of epileptogenesis and for the discovery and the trial design of antiepileptogenic agents (14).

References

1. **Sillanpää M, Schmidt D.** Epilepsy: long-term rates of childhood-onset epilepsy remission confirmed. *Nat Rev Neurol* 2015; **11**(3):130–131.
2. **Shorvon SD, Goodridge DM.** Longitudinal cohort studies of the prognosis of epilepsy: contribution of the National General Practice Study of Epilepsy and other studies. *Brain* 2013; **136**(Pt 11):3497–3510.
3. **Sillanpää M, Saarinen M, Schmidt D.** Clinical conditions of long-term cure in childhood-onset epilepsy: a 45-year follow-up study. *Epilepsy Behav* 2014; **37**:49–53.
4. **Braun KP, Schmidt D.** Stopping antiepileptic drugs in seizure-free patients. *Curr Opin Neurol* 2014; **27**(2):219–226.
5. **Medical Research Council Antiepileptic Drug Withdrawal Study Group.** Randomised study of antiepileptic drug withdrawal in patients in remission. *Lancet* 1991; **337**(8751):1175–1180.
6. **Löscher W, Klitgaard H, Twyman RE, Schmidt D.** New avenues for anti-epileptic drug discovery and development. *Nat Rev Drug Discov* 2013; **12**(10):757–776.
7. **Löscher W, Klotz U, Zimprich F, Schmidt D.** The clinical impact of pharmacogenetics on the treatment of epilepsy. *Epilepsia* 2009; **50**(1):1–23.
8. **Easterford K, Clough P, Comish S, Lawton L, Duncan S.** The use of complementary medicines and alternative practitioners in a cohort of patients with epilepsy. *Epilepsy Behav* 2005; **6**(1):59–62.
9. **Doering JH, Reuner G, Kadish NE, Pietz J, Schubert-Bast S.** Pattern and predictors of complementary and alternative medicine (CAM) use among pediatric patients with epilepsy. *Epilepsy Behav* 2013; **29**(1):41–46.
10. **Zaccara G, Giovannelli F, Schmidt D.** Placebo and nocebo responses in drug trials of epilepsy. *Epilepsy Behav* 2015; **43**:128–134.
11. **Kaptchuk TJ, Miller FG.** Placebo effects in medicine. *N Engl J Med* 2015; **373**(1):8–9.

12. **Avorn J, Kesselheim AS.** The 21st century cures act—will it take us back in time? *N Engl J Med* 2015; **372**(26):2473–2475.
13. **Schmidt D.** Is antiepileptogenesis a realistic goal in clinical trials? Concerns and new horizons. *Epileptic Disord* 2012; **14**(2):105–113.
14. **Löscher W, Hirsch LJ, Schmidt D.** The enigma of the latent period in the development of symptomatic acquired epilepsy—traditional view versus new concepts. *Epilepsy Behav* 2015; **52**(Pt A):78–92.

Appendix

Dating Epilepsy

In this final section, we list the dates of important events in the narrative of clinical epilepsy in the era which is the topic of our book (Table A.1). In constructing this list, we have followed various rules: we have not mentioned by name anyone still living; we have included the dates of publication of books which we feel are of great importance and in doing so have introduced our own selective bias; we have included the dates of introduction of antiepileptic drugs still on the formulary but not the very many which were introduced and then subsequently withdrawn or which have fallen from use; we have included the dates of the first publication or presentation of surgical procedures for epilepsy although these were usually developed in a period prior to first publication; and we have included only those surgical operations still practised. We have not listed the dates of introduction of new investigatory, surgical, or treatment technologies, as these were usually not specifically invented for epilepsy (but have given some detail of these in the endnote[1]); we have other events but not dates of importance in experimental epilepsy.

Table A.1 Chronology of key moments in the study of epilepsy (1857–present)

1857	Effect of potassium bromide on epilepsy first reported by Sir Charles Locock (1799–1875), a chance discovery which opened a new era of therapy for epilepsy
1859	The National Hospital for the Cure and Relief of Paralysis and Epilepsy, was established in London as the first hospital devoted to the treatment of epilepsy. Around this time too, a number of epilepsy 'colonies' were established for care and employment, e.g. Bielefeld-Bethel (Germany, 1867), La Teppe (France, 1857), Heemstede (Netherlands,1882), Chalfont (England, 1893), Zurich (Switzerland, 1886), Gallapolis (Ohio, USA, 1891), Craig Colony (Sonyea, New York, USA, 1896), Dianalund (Denmark, 1897), Kork (Germany, 1892), Quarriers (Scotland, 1906), and Sandvika (Norway, 1911).
1861	Sir John Russell Reynolds (1828–1896), a physician in London, was arguably the first to consider in his 1861 treatise on epilepsy that an idiopathic disease, epilepsy, existed, one to be distinguished from 'epileptiform' seizures due to brain pathology.

1870	The physiologist Fritsch (1838–1927) and psychiatrist Hitzig (1838–1907) publish *On the Electric Excitability of the Cerebrum* (1870) in which they provoked seizures by electric stimulation in the brain cortex of dogs
1873	Publication of *Study of Convulsions*; in 1873 by Sir John Hughlings Jackson (1835–1911) defined epilepsy: 'Epilepsy is the name for occasional, sudden, excessive, rapid and local discharges of grey matter'. Jean-Martin Charcot (1825–1893) coined the term Jacksonian seizures, a type of focal seizures with preserved consciousness
1881	Publication of first edition of *Epilepsy and Other Chronic Convulsive Disorders* by Sir William Gowers (1845–1915), a physician in London, which was a landmark in the history of epilepsy
1886	Sir Victor Horsley carries out first cortical resective surgery for epilepsy, an operation which opened the modern era of epilepsy surgery
1887	Paraldehyde used for epilepsy (the drug was entered into the formulary in 1874)
1903	Hermann Bernhard Lundborg (1868–1943), a Swedish physician, notorious for his views on eugenics, published his research on the genetics of what was later called Unverricht–Lundborg disease, a progressive myoclonic epilepsy first described by Heinrich Unverricht in 1891 (1853–1912)
1904	Publication of *Epilepsy and its Treatment* by William Spratling (1863–1915), the first major textbook on epilepsy published in the United States
1907	*The Borderlands of Epilepsy* was published focusing on syncope, migraine, vertigo, and narcolepsy by Sir William Gowers (1845–1915) Indiana becomes the first US state to enact a eugenic compulsory sterilisation law for people with mental deficiency and included patients with epilepsy Publication of *Epilepsy – A Study of the Idiopathic Disease* by W. Aldren Turner (1864–1945)
1909	The International League Against Epilepsy (ILAE) was established in Budapest on August 30 1909. Launch of first series of *Epilepsia* which continued publication until 1914
1911	First publication of fasting as a therapy for epilepsy in the modern era (by Guelpa and Marie) which was a prelude to the ketogenic diet
1912	The effect of phenobarbital on epilepsy reported for the first time by Alfred Hauptmann (1881–1948) in Freiburg, Germany
1914	ILAE ceases activities with the outbreak of the First World War. It was formed again in 1935, then again ceased activities in the Second World War and resumed its work in 1945.
1921	Russell Wilder (1885–1959) at the Mayo Clinic describes the first trial of the ketogenic diet
1923	Walter Dandy (1886–1946) carries out the first hemispherectomy in a human patient
1924	Hans Berger (1873–1941) records the first human EEG (reported in 1929) Publication of the first edition (in Dutch) of L. J. J. Muskens' book *Epilepsy: Comparative Pathogenesis, Symptoms and Treatment*

1926	Intravenous phenobarbital reported to be used in status epilepticus
1927	*Buck* v *Bell* case in US supreme court rules in favour of forced sterilisation of epileptic patients
1929	Berger published first human EEG
1931	Dandy carries out the first corpus callosal section to remove a congenital cyst
1934	Adrian and Matthews publish a renowned paper in *Brain* corroborating Berger's EEG findings
1935	Gibbs, Davis, and Lennox describe the interictal spike waves and the 3/sec pattern of absence seizures The first intraoperative electrocorticogram by Foerster and Altenburger A group of neurologists meet at Lingfield Epilepsy Centre and relaunch the ILAE
1936	First clinical EEG laboratory set up at Massachusetts General Hospital
1937	Second series of *Epilepsia* launched and continued publication until 1950
1938	First reports of the use of phenytoin by Merritt (1902–1979) and Putnam (1894–1975) using the maximal electroshock method of screening in cats
1939	Action T4—the mass murder of handicapped persons with epilepsy begins in Nazi Germany
1940	The first corpus callosectomy for epilepsy is reported by van Wagenen and Herren
1941	Frederic Andrews Gibbs (1903–1992) and Erna Leonhardt-Gibbs (1904–1987) established the correlation between EEG findings and epileptic seizures around this time, and publish the *Atlas of Electroencephalography* with William Lennox (1884–1960) Acetazolamide (Diamox; Lederle) introduced for the treatment of epilepsy
1948	Around this time, the first temporal lobectomy with removal of the mesial structures is performed, by either Arthur Morris in Georgetown or Wilder Penfield (1891–1976) in Montreal
1952	Third series of *Epilepsia* launched and ceased publication in 1955
1953	Introduction of the EEG as a guide to perform temporal lobe surgery by Bailey and Gibbs in 1953.
1954	*Epilepsy and the Functional Anatomy of the Human Brain* published by Wilder Penfield (1891–1976), and Herbert Jasper (1906–1999) Primidone (Mysoline; ICI) introduced into clinical practice
1956	Intravenous phenytoin first used in status epilepticus
1957	Jean Talairach (1911–2007) a neurosurgeon at the Centre Hospitalier Ste. Anne in Paris, published a stereotactic atlas. The term stereoelectroencephalography (SEEG) was introduced in 1962 by Talairach and Jean Bancaud (1921–1993)
1958	Ethosuximide (Zarontin; Parke, Davis) reported to be effective by R. Vossen

1959	First edition of *Basic Mechanisms of the Epilepsies* published by J. Kiffin Penry (1929–1996) Fourth series of *Epilepsia* launched and continues to be published
1960	Publication of *Epilepsy and Related Disorders* by William Lennox and his daughter Margaret Lennox
1961	The International Bureau for Epilepsy (IBE) was established as an organisation of laypersons and professionals interested in the medical and non-medical aspects of epilepsy
1963	Kefauver–Harris amendments to FDA regulations Benzodiazepines, in the form of diazepam and chlordiazepoxide, introduced into clinical practice and diazepam also used in status epilepticus Discovery of valproate reported by H. Meunier, G. Carraz, and Y. Meunier
1964	Henri Gastaut (1915–1995) produces the first draft of the ILAE Classification of Seizure Type
1965	Carbamazepine introduced into the market in Britain and within a few years is other countries in Europe Talairach, Bancaud and co-workers publish *La stéréoélectroencéphalographie dans l'épilepsie*
1966	First randomised trial of carbamazepine published Epilepsy section formed at NIH with J. Kiffin Penry as chief
1967	Valproate (Epilim; Sanofi) approved for use first in France
1968	Clonazepam (Rivotril; Roche) licensed for treatment of epilepsy in Europe
1969	ILAE Classification of Seizure Type presented to the General Assembly of the ILAE in New York. Henri Gastaut described the Lennox–Gastaut syndrome *Basic Mechanisms of the Epilepsies* published by H. H. Jasper, A. A. Ward, and A. Pope
1970	Establishment of the ILAE Commission on Antiepileptic Drugs
1971	Gastaut reported excellent results of intravenous clonazepam in status epilepticus
1972	First edition of *Antiepileptic Drugs* by D. M. Woodbury, J. K. Penry, and R. P. Schmidt published (the fifth and last edition was published in 2002)
1975	Clobazam (Frisium; Roche) licensed in Europe for the treatment of epilepsy J. Kiffin Penry, with Harvey Kupferberg and Ewart Swinyard establish the Antiepileptic Drug Development Program at NIH
1953	Murray Falconer (1910–1977) introduced the en bloc anterior temporal lobe resection and the term mesial temporal sclerosis.
1978	Antimyoclonic effect of piracetam (Nootropil; UCB) demonstrated First published reports of the advantages of antiepileptic drug monotherapy —and the beginning of the 'monotherapy age' Publication of Commission for the Control of Epilepsy and Its Consequences. *Plan for Nationwide Action in Epilepsy* by the US government

1981	Revision of the ILAE Classification of Epileptic Seizures approved
1982	Morrell and Whisler report the first case treated by multiple subpial transection First investigations of SPECT scanning in epilepsy Clinical MRI introduced and first large published series of neurological patients some with epilepsy
1989	Introduction of 'third-generation drugs' begins initially with vigabatrin (Sabril; Marion Merrill Dow) in Europe and zonisamide in Japan (Excegran; Dianippon)
1990	Lamotrigine (Lamictal; Burroughs-Wellcome) licensed first in Ireland and a year later in the United Kingdom
1990	Oxcarbazepine (Trileptal; Novartis) licensed first in Denmark, and then in the European Union generally in 1999 and in the United States in 2000
1992	First biannual Eilat Conference on New Antiepileptic Drugs held
1993	Felbamate (Felbatrol; Carter-Wallace) licensed in the United States, but not in Europe, and then rapidly withdrawn
1994	Gabapentin (Neurontin; Parke-Davis) licensed in the United States and United Kingdom
1995	Topiramate (Topamax; Johnson and Johnson) licensed in the United Kingdom and subsequently widely in Europe and the United States First 'epilepsy gene' published
1996	Tiagabine (Gabatril: Novo-Nordisk) licensed first in France and then widely in Europe and the United States
1996	Cochrane epilepsy group registered in the Cochrane collaboration
1997	Launch of the Global Campaign Against Epilepsy (Out of the Shadows) Vagal nerve stimulation receives a US regulatory approval as a treatment for partial-onset epilepsy
1999	Levetiracetam (Keppra; UCB) licensed as a treatment for epilepsy in the United States and in Europe a year later
2004	Pregabalin (Lyrica; Pfizer) licensed in Europe for epilepsy
2004	Buccal midazolam (as midazolam maleate (Epistatus; Special Products) permitted under special licence in the United Kingdom
2007	Stiripentol (Diacomit; Biocodex) licensed for use in SMEI in Europe
2007	Rufinamide (Inovelon (Europe) and Banzel (United States); Eisai) licensed for use in Lennox–Gastaut Syndrome in Europe
2008	Lacosamide (Vimpat; UCB) licensed in Europe, and in the United States in 2009
2010	Retigabine (ezogabine) (Trobalt; GlaxoSmithKline in Europe, and Potiga; Valeant in United States) licensed in 2010 in United States and 2011 in Europe EMA approval for Medronics Deep Brain Stimulation Therapy for treatment of epilepsy

Table A.1 Continued

2011	Buccal midazolam in the form of midazolam hydrochloride (Buccolam; Viropharma) licensed in Europe under PUMA scheme
2012	Perampanel (Trobalt; Eisai) licensed in Europe and United States in 2012 EMA approval for NeuroSigma external Trigeminal Nerve Stimulation (eTNS) system in epilepsy
2013	Publication of seizure prediction studies using implanted Neurovista device NeuroPace RNS stimulator approved by FDA for treatment of epilepsy

Source: data from Magiorkinis E, Diamantis A, Sidiropoulou K, and Panteliadis C. Highlights in the history of epilepsy: the last 200 years. *Epilepsy Research and Treatment*, Volume 2014, Article ID 582039, Copyright © 2014 Emmanouil Magiorkinis et al.; Shorvon SD, Weiss G, Avanzini G, Engel P, Meinardi H, Moshe S, et al. (2009) *International League Against Epilepsy 1909–2009: A Centenary History*. Oxford: Wiley Blackwell, Copyright © 2009 John Wiley and Sons; Shorvon SD. Historical Introduction. In: Shorvon SD, Dreifuss F, Fish D, and Thomas D (eds). *The Treatment of Epilepsy*, 1st edition. Oxford: Blackwell Science Ltd., Copyright © 1996 Blackwell Science Ltd.; Shorvon SD. Historical Introduction. In: Shorvon SD, Dodson E, Fish DR, and Perucca E (eds). *The Treatment of Epilepsy*, 2nd edition. Oxford: Blackwell Science Ltd.; Shorvon SD. Historical Introduction. In: Shorvon SD, Perucca E, and Engel J (eds). *The Treatment of Epilepsy*, 3rd edition. Oxford: Wiley-Blackwell, Copyright © 2009 Wiley-Blackwell Ltd.; Shorvon SD. Historical Introduction. In: Shorvon SD, Perucca E, Engel J, *The Treatment of Epilepsy*, 4th edition. Oxford: Wiley-Blackwell, Copyright © 2015 John Wiley and Sons, Ltd.; Shorvon SD, Weiss G, Wolf P, and Andermann F (eds.). Special Issue: Aspects of the history of epilepsy 1909–2009. *Epilepsia*, Volume 50, Supplement 3, Copyright © 2009 International League Against Epilepsy.

Note

1. Investigatory modalities introduced into neurology in general but which were to prove of great importance for epilepsy included air ventriculography introduced in 1918 by Walter Dandy; cerebral angiography in 1926 by Igas Moniz; depth EEG first reported in 1962; CT scanning, invented by Godfrey Hounsfield, introduced into clinical epilepsy practice in 1972; the first MRI scanner was constructed in Nottingham by Peter Mansfield in 1976 and the first large series in epilepsy in 1982; first report of PET scanning in epilepsy in 1978; first SPECT scan reported in a patient with epilepsy in 1982; and first series of magnetic resonance spectroscopy in epilepsy in 1984. Other events in the history of drug treatment which were to have an important impact in epilepsy include the first randomised controlled trial published in 1948, of streptomycin, and the Cochrane Collaboration which was formed in 1972. Trial registration was introduced in 2004 by the International Committee of Medical Journal Editors. Surgical developments introduced into neurosurgery, and which were to have an important impact in epilepsy, included the introduction of the operating microscope in 1957, the gamma knife by Leksell in 1968, and linear accelerator (Linac)-based neurosurgery in 1985.

Index

Abbreviations used in the index can be found in the table on page xiii.
Page numbers suffixed with *f* refer to material in figures, *t* tables and *b* boxes

absence seizures, valproate, 53
access, medical journals/publishing, 141–3
acetazolamide (Diamox), 175t
adhesive personality, 24
adjunctive treatments, 116
Adrian, Edgar Douglas, 87, 104, 175t
aetiology of epilepsy *see* causes (aetiology) of epilepsy
aggressiveness, post-temporal lobectomy, 100–1
air encephalography, 87
air ventriculography, 87, 104
alternative and complementary medicine, 163–4
 drug interactions, 164
AMPA receptors, 63f
anaesthesia, 81–2
 developments in, 92
Andruszkiewicz, Ryszard, 75
angiography, 104
animal extracts, antiepileptic drugs, 40–1, 41t
animal models
 causes of epilepsy, 133
 clinical trials, 111
anterior temporal lobe resection, 175t
antidepressants, 111
antiepileptic drugs, 39–60
 additional clinical value, 77–8
 adverse effects, 162
  behavioural changes *see* behaviour changes
  depression *see* depression
  long-term, 156–7
 animal extracts, 40–1, 41t
 blood concentration measurement, 64
 clinical testing *see* clinical testing/trials
 combination therapy, 162
 costs of, 118
 discontinuation, 156
 discover and development, pharmaceutical company development, 57–8
 discovery and development, 54, 158–67, 160–1t
  biomarkers, 112, 167–8
  cost of, 54, 150
  difficulties, 163
  future targets, 159f
  genetic testing, 112
  identification failure, 112
  improved effectiveness, 112–13
  molecular biology, 57–8
  pharmaceutical company development, 54
  pharmacogenic alterations, 170
  pharmacogenomics, 57–8
  random screening, 112
  repurposing existing drugs, 159
  structural variants, 112
  target-based drug design, 112, 158–9
  trial-and-error, 112
  valid targets, 167
  see also clinical testing/trials
 efficacy differentiation, 77
 history of, vi
  1940, 45b
  1955, 49–50b
  1960s to present, 61–80
  1996-2004, 55–6t
  future work, 158f, 166–7
  introduction through time, 67f
 mechanisms of action, 63f, 112
 multitarget treatments (pleotherapy), 159
 new (novel) drugs, 108
 old (classic) drugs, 108
 patient subsets, 162
 plant derivatives, 40–1, 41t
 in pregnancy, 108
 prescription of, 151–2
 professional organisations, 61–5
 regulation, 54, 57–8
 single-target treatments, 159
 to specific types of epilepsy, 162–3
Antiepileptic Drugs (Woodbury et al), 64, 176t
antiepileptogenesis, 167–8
antisepsis, 104
 surgery, 81
Aping Mankind (Tallis), 134
artificial demand of surgery, 102
asylums, 22
atavism, 26
 causes of epilepsy, 129–30
Atlas of Electroencephalography (Lennox), 175t
authorship of papers, 141
auto-intoxication, 130
awake craniotomy, 89
Ayurveda pills, drug interactions, 164

Bailey, Percival, 87
barbiturates, 48–9, 49b
　mechanism of action, 63f
Basic Mechanisms of the Epilepsies, 176t
Bateson, William, 18
Bayesian methods in clinical trial
　　design, 165–6
Beck, Adolf, 86
behaviour changes
　levetiracetam (Keppra), 71
　post-surgery, 100–1
　temporal lobectomy, 99
　temporal lobes, 98
belladonna, 43, 46
benzodiazepines, 48–9, 53–4, 66
　discovery, 178t
　introduction, 50
　mechanism of action, 63f
Berger, Hans, 86–7, 104, 175t
Berlin Declaration on Open Access to
　　Knowledge in the Sciences and
　　Humanities, 142
La Bête Humaine (Zola), 26, 28f
Bethel Colony (Germany), 22, 29
Bethesda Statement of Open Access, 142
Bialer, Meir, 62
biomarkers, 112, 167–8
black swan, 79
Blackwell's Island (USA), 22
blood concentration measurement,
　　antiepileptic drugs, 64
borax, 43, 46
The Borderlands of Epilepsy (Gowers), 174t
"botanical" classification of
　　epilepsy, 16–17
Brain Rescue, 136
brain stimulation, 93–4
brilliant red dye, 46
brivaracetam, 69, 112
bromaline, 42
bromapin, 42
bromide
　adverse effects, 42–3
　development of, 42–4
　formulations used, 42
　introduction, 39
　Locock, Charles, 41
bromism, 42–3
bromoderma, 43
Budapest Open Access Initiative, 142

Cairns, Hugh, 89
calcium channel blockade, 58
　drug mechanisms, 63f
carbamazepine, 54, 66
　advantages, 52
　advertisement, 51f
　discovery, 178t

introduction, 39, 50, 52
　mechanism of action, 63f
　progabide co-medication, 78
carisbamate, 112
Catel, Werner, 37
Caton, Richard, 86
causes (aetiology) of epilepsy, 127–35
　atavism, 129–30
　auto-intoxication, 130
　cellular mechanisms, 6
　central nervous system developmental
　　defects, 26
　criminality, 130
　in definition, 7
　evolution over time, 8
　heredity linked to theory of
　　degeneration, 129–30
　Jackson, 127–8
　Lennox, 128–9, 128f, 129f
　level of, 7–8
　molecular biology, 133
　molecular genetics, 132
　neurological taint, 129–30
　psychoanalysis, 130–1
　structural abnormalities, 131–2
cellular mechanisms, seizures, 6
central nervous system (CNS), developmental
　　defects, 26
cerebral cortex, 86
　functional maps, 83
cerebral localisation, 82–3
Chalfont (UK), 22
characteristic (epileptic) personality, 24
Charcot, Jean-Marie, 17, 84–5, 174t
chemical nature of seizures, 6–7
children, resolution of seizures, 155–6
China, attitudes to epilepsy, 35
chloral hydrate, 43
chlordiazepoxide, 176t
chloroform, 81
chronic seizure tests, 112
citations, 140
Clark, Leon Pierce, 24–5
classifications of epilepsy, 12–17
　botanical classification, 16–17
　"botanical" classification of epilepsy, 16–17
　drug-resistant epilepsy (refractory epilepsy)
　　see drug-resistant epilepsy (refractory
　　epilepsy)
　focal self-limited epilepsy syndrome, 156f
　gardener's classification, 13
　idiopathic epilepsies, 132–3
　idiopathic generalised epilepsy *see*
　　idiopathic generalised epilepsy
　idiopathic partial epilepsy, 132–3
　limbic epilepsy (temporal lobe
　　epilepsy), 95–6
　seizures type, 13

temporal lobe epilepsy (limbic epilepsy), 95–6
uncharacterised epilepsy, 156f
uncomplicated epilepsy, 156f
clinically irrelevant controls in clinical trials, 112–13
clinical testing/trials, 57, 110–18
  analysis errors, 121–2
  animal tests, 111
  benefits, 118
  business enterprises, 117–18
  clinically irrelevant controls, 112–13
  clinical value of data, 114–15
  credibility of, 121
  criticism of statistics, 135
  heterogeneity of disease, 115
  low clinical value end points, 115–16
  monotherapy trials, 117
  non-traditional designs, 165–6
  numbers needed, 111–12
  placebo delay, 114
  seizure frequency, 110–11
  size and cost, 115
clobazam (Frisium), 109, 176t
clonazepam (Rivotril), 176t
cognitive changes, post-surgery, 100–1
colonies, 22, 175t
commercial environment, fraud, 124
Commission on Antiepileptic Drugs, ILAE, 145, 178t
Commission on Classification and Terminology, ILAE, 145
commissions, ILAE, 145
Community Patients Transport Service, 31–2
co-morbid diseases, 109
complete remission, long-term studies, 155, 156f
computed tomography (CT), 92
  causes of epilepsy, 131
  overuse of, 119
concealment of symptoms, 26, 28
concept of disability, 10–11
conferences, ILAE, 144
congruence, concept of, 94–5
constipation, 43–4
Cook, Mark, 111
corpus callosectomy, 91, 175t
cortical resections, surgery, 86
Corton, Henry, 130
criminality, 25t, 130
CT *see* computed tomography (CT)
Cushing, Harvey, 85–6

Dandy, Walter, 87, 104–5, 174t, 175t
  corpus callosectomy, 91
  hemispherectomy, 90
data, falsified, 123–4
Davenport, Charles B, 29

deep brain stimulation (DBS), 93
defensive attitudes, 35
definitions of epilepsy, 7–11
  causes, 7
  concept of disability, 10–11
  genetics, 9–10
  ILAE, 11–12
  medical perspective, 16
  non-medical approaches, 11
  societal perspective, 16
degeneracy, inherited, 24
degeneration, theories of, 21–6, 129–30
Delasiauve, Louis, 39–40
demonic possession, 21, 22
dependency, phenobarbital, 45
depression, 109
  drug-resistant epilepsy, 108
developing countries, 110
Diacomit (stiripentol), 162, 177t
Diamox (acetazolamide), 177t
diazepam, 178t
disability, concept of, 10–11
disturbed mental states, 24
Dravet syndrome, 162
Dreifuss, Fritz E, 13, 18, 46, 62
drug regulation, 54, 57–8, 149–52
  changes in, 78
  guidelines, 150–1
  medical quality evaluation, 151
drug-resistant epilepsy (refractory epilepsy), 107–10, 168
  criteria for, 107–8
  depression, 108
  future targets and treatments, 159f
  mechanisms, 108, 158–9
  monotherapy trials, 117
  premature mortality, 108–9

economic burden of epilepsy, 110
EEG *see* electroencephalography (EEG)
Eilat conferences, 62, 160–1t
electrical stimulation, surgery, 86
electroencephalography (EEG)
  adverse effects, 118–19
  causes of epilepsy, 132
  classification of epilepsy, 13
  development, 89–90
  discovery, 5–6, 175t
  history of, 86–8, 87f
  intracranial, 89–90
  overuse of, 119
  video-telemetry, 90
EMA *see* European Medicines Agency (EMA)
emotional changes, post-surgery, 100–1
emotional poverty, 131
'en bloc temporal lobe' resection, 89
enforced sterilisation, 30
Engel Jr., Jerome, 62
environmental factors, 132–3

epidemiology of epilepsy, v–vi
Epilepsia, 136, 137f, 138, 144–5
    first printing, 174t
    growth of, 138f
Epilepsia Open, 144
Epilepsy and Behavior, 138
Epilepsy and its Treatment (Spratling), 174t
Epilepsy and Other Chronic Convulsive Disorders (Gowers), 174t
Epilepsy and Related Disorders (Lennox), 176t
Epilepsy and the Functional Anatomy of the Human Brain (Penfield), 88–9, 175t
Epilepsy: A Study of the Idiopathic Disease (Turner), 58, 174t
epilepsy colonies, 22, 173t
Epilepsy: Comparative Pathogenesis, Symptoms and Treatment (Muskens), 174t
Epilepsy International, 148
Epilepsy Journal, 136, 138
Epileptic Disorders, 138, 144
epileptic wards, 22
epileptogenic zone, 95, 96
Epistatus (midazolam), 177t, 178t
eslicarbazepine acetate, 63f
ethosuximide (Zarontin), 47, 50, 63f, 175t
eugenics, 29–34
    enforced sterilisation, 30
    Human Genetics, 32–3
    marriage prevention, 30, 33
    Nazis, 31–2, 32f, 175t
    scientific principles, 30–1
    sterilization, 175t
Eugenics Record Office, 29
European Medicines Agency (EMA), 150
    clinical trials, 117
Excegran (zonisamide), 63f, 177t
Eymard, P, 52
ezogabine (retigabine/Trobalt), 63f, 112, 163, 177t

Falconer, Murray, 89, 176t
The Falling Sickness (Temkin), 2f, vii
falsified data, 122–3
family support, 35
Fariello, Ruggero, 62
FDA *see* Food and Drug Administration (FDA)
felbamate (Felbatrol), 163–4, 177t
Ferrier, David, 3f, 82–3
financial considerations, surgery, 101
fMRI *see* functional magnetic resonance imaging (fMRI)
focal seizures, 5
focal self-limited epilepsy syndrome, 156f
Foerster, Otfrid, 86, 175t
follow-ups, long-term, 116–17

Food and Drug Administration (FDA)
    drug approval, 75, 114
    formation, 149
    functions, 149–50
    regulatory powers, 57
fraud, 122–5
    commercial environment, 124
    falsified data, 122–4
    medical journals/publishing, 141
    misleading by patients, 124–5
    Munchausen syndrome by proxy, 124–5
Frisium (clobazam), 109, 176t
Fritsch, Gustav, 82, 174t
frontal lobectomy, 99
frontal lobotomy, 99, 101
functional hemispherectomy, 90–1
functional magnetic resonance imaging (fMRI), 93, 105
    causes of epilepsy, 134
functional maps, cerebral cortex, 83

gabapentin (Neurontin), 61, 66, 73–5
    introduction, 177t
    mechanism of action, 63f, 74
    phase II clinical studies, 74
GABA receptors
    antiepileptic drug mechanisms, 112–13
    blocking of, 58
    drug mechanisms, 63f
    gabapentin (Neurontin) mechanism, 74
    phenobarbital mechanism, 48
Gabatril (tiagabine), 109, 112, 177t
Galton, Francis, 29, 39
gardener's classification, 13
Gastaut, Henri Jean Pascal, 13, 14f, 18, 176t
Gawande, Atul, 119
Gélineau's formula, 42
generalised seizures, partial seizures *vs.*, 5
generalized anxiety disorder, 109
Genes, Cells and Brains (Rose & Rose), 134–5
genetics, definition of epilepsy, 9–10
genetic testing, 112
Germany, attitudes to epilepsy, 35
Gibbs, Frederic Andrew, 176t
Global Campaign Against Epilepsy (Out of the Shadows), 146, 147f, 179t
glutamanergic excitation, 112–13
Godlee, Rickman, 82, 104
Goffman, Irving, 34
Goltz, Friedrich Leopold, 82–3
Gower, Alma J, 68
Gowers, William, 3f, 167–8, 174t
Gram, Lennart, 64

Haeckel, Ernst, 129–30
Hallervorden, Julius, 11, 18

Harcourt, Vernon, 81
Hauptmann, Alfred, 44, 174t
hemispherectomy, 90-1, 174t
Hereditary Courts, 31
heterogeneity of disease in clinical
    trials, 115
Heyde, Werner, 37
Hindu Marriage Act 1955 (India), 33
hippocampectomy of Yaşargil, 92
Hitzig, Eduard, 82, 176t
Holmes, Oliver Wendell, 1, 30, 33
Hönack, Doris, 78-9
Horsley, Victor, 3f, 81, 82, 84f, 85f, 174t
    functional brain maps, 83
Hounsfield, Godfrey Newbold, 105
Human Genetics, eugenics, 32-3
human identity, 10
human rights, 10
    societal attitudes, 34
hydantoins, 48-9, 49-50b
hydrobromic acid, 42

IBE see International Bureau for
    Epilepsy (IBE)
ictal onset zone, 95
idiopathic epilepsies, 132-3
idiopathic generalised epilepsy, 7
    genetic causes, 132-3
    valproate, 53
idiopathic partial epilepsy, 132-3
ILAE see International League Against
    Epilepsy (ILAE)
Illich, Ivan, 9
impact factor (IF), 139-40
indexing, 142-3
inherited degeneracy, 24
Inovelon (rufinamide), 177t
interictal abnormalities, 6
International Bureau for Epilepsy (IBE)
    establishment, 178t
    ILAE, relationship with, 148
International Committee of Medical Journal
    Editors, 152
International Congress of Neurology, 15f
International League Against Epilepsy
    (ILAE), 62, 64
    achievements, 146-7
    bureaucracy in, 143-9
    change in structure, 146-8
    chapters of, 143
    classifications of epilepsy, 12-17, 177t
        drug-resistant epilepsy, 107-8
    classifications of seizure type, 176t
    Commission on Antiepileptic Drugs, 64,
        145, 176t
    Commission on Classification and
        Terminology, 145
    commissions, 145

conferences, 144
definitions of epilepsy, 11-12
finances, 145-6, 145f
foundation, 143, 174t
functions, 144
Global Campaign Against Epilepsy,
    146, 147f
International Bureau for Epilepsy (IBE),
    relationship with, 148
journal management, 136
    see also Epilepsia
pharmaceutical industry role, 148-9
publications, 144
taskforces, 145
    Task Force on Classification and
        Terminology, 15-16
intracranial brain stimulation, 93-4
irritative zone, 95
isotope scanning, 134

Jacksonian seizures, 5
Jackson, John Hughlings, 3f, 174t
    causes of epilepsy, 127-8
    cerebral localisation, 82
    classifications of epilepsy, 12-13
    definition of epilepsy, 7
    seizure definitions, 1, 3, 5
    temporal lobe seizures, 86
Jasper, Herbert, 88-9, 175t
Jelliffe, Smith Ely, 131
Joannidis, John, 135
John, Prince, 26, 28
Journal of Epilepsy, 138
journals see medical journals/publishing

KCNQ potassium channel, 63f
Kefauver-Harris Amendment, 149
Keppra see levetiracetam (Keppra)
ketogenic diet, 174t
Keytruda, 166
Klitgaard, Henrik, 69
Krause, Fedor, 86
Krynauw, Rowland Anthony, 90, 105

lacosamide (Vimpat), 63f, 177t
lamotrigine (Lamictal), 61, 66, 71-2
    introduction, 177t
    mechanism of action, 63f
lamotrigine-resistant kindled rat, 112
The Lancet, 135
Leber, Paul, 117
Lennox-Gastault syndrome, 162, 176t
Lennox, William Gordon, 17, 175t, 176t
    causes of epilepsy, 128-9, 128f, 129f
    definition of epilepsy, 7
    eugenics, 33
Leonhardt-Gibbs, Erna, 175t
lesionectomy, 93

levetiracetam (Keppra), 61, 66, 68–74
  adverse effects, 70
  commercial release, 69–70
  depression, 109
  development, 78–9
  generic manufacturing, 70
  introduction, 68
  licensing, 177t
  marketing, 70–1
  mechanism of action, 63f, 69
  physician preference, 70
Levy, René, 62
limbic epilepsy (temporal lobe
  epilepsy), 95–6
Lister, Joseph, 39, 81, 104
Lloyd, Kenneth, 62
Locock, Charles, 41, 173t
Lombroso, Cesare, 25–6, 37
long-term adverse effects of antiepileptic
  drugs, 156–7
long-term epilepsy cure, 169–70
long-term follow-ups, 116–17
long-term studies of complete remission,
  155, 156f
long-term treatment, 120
Löscher, Wolfgang, 64–5, 68–9, 78–9
low-value care, 118–21
Lundborg, Hermann Bernhard, 174t
Lyrica *see* pregabalin (Lyrica)

Macewen, William, 81, 82
magnetic resonance imaging (MRI), 92–3
  causes of epilepsy, 131
  guided stereotaxy, 93–4
  introduction, 177t
  overuse of, 119
magneto-encephalography, 134
marriage prevention, 30, 33
Matthews, BHC, 87, 175t
maximal electric shock (MES), 68, 111
medical journals/publishing, 122, 135–43
  access, 141–3
  authorship of papers, 141
  citations, 140
  difficulties of articles of value, 139–40
  fraud, 141
  ILAE, 144
  impact factor (IF), 139–40
  indexing, 142–3
  numbers of, 135–6
    disadvantages, 139
  peer reviews, 140–1
  profits in, 139
  publication record, 141
  reviews, 140
  substandard, 139
  validity of, 140–1
  value of, 136

worldwide web effect, 138–9
medical model of epilepsy, 9
medical perspective, definition of epilepsy, 16
Medline (PubMed), 142–3
Medronic Deep Brain Stimulation
  Therapy, 177t
Mellick, Larry B, 74
memory, temporal lobes, 98
mental handicaps, association with
  epilepsy, 34
mental states, disturbed, 24
Merritt, H Houston, 47, 177t
MES (maximal electric shock), 68, 111
mesial temporal sclerosis, 176t
methyl blue dye, 46
Meunier, H, 52
Meunier, Y, 52
midazolam (Epistatus), 177t, 178t
migraine, 73
misdiagnosis of epilepsy, 120, 157
misleading by patients, 124–5
Molaison, Henry, 105
molecular biology
  antiepileptic drugs, 57–8
  causes of epilepsy, 133
molecular genetics
  causes of epilepsy, 132
  definition of epilepsy, 9–10
Moniz, Egas, 99, 105
monotherapy trials, 117
mood effects
  lamotrigine (Lamictal), 72
  temporal lobes, 98
Morel, Bénédict Augustin, 23–4, 37
Morrell procedure (multiple subpial
  transection), 91–2, 178t
Morris, Arthur, 88, 175t
Morselli, Paolo, 62
mortality
  premature, 108–9
  from surgery, 98
MRI *see* magnetic resonance imaging (MRI)
multiple subpial transection (Morrell
  procedure), 91–2, 177t
multitarget treatments (pleotherapy), 159
Munchausen syndrome by proxy, 124–5
Muskens, LJJ, 174t
myoclonic seizures, 53
Mysoline (primidone), 175t

National General Practice Study on
  Epilepsy, 169
National Hospital for the Paralysed and
  Epileptic, 83–5
National Hospital for the Relief and Cure of the
  Paralysed and the Epileptic, 3f, 173t
National Institute for Health and Care
  Excellence (NICE), 151

National Institute of Health (NIH), 176t
National Institute of Mental Health (NIMH), 72
National Institute of Neurological Disorders and Stroke (NINDS), 64
Nazi Germany, 31–2, 32f, 175t
Neurological Trait
  attitudes to epilepsy, 24
  causes of epilepsy, 129–30
neuronal networks, 133
Neurontin *see* gabapentin (Neurontin)
neuropathic taint, eugenics, 30
neurosurgery *see* surgery
neurotoxic effects, phenobarbital, 45
new (novel) antiepileptic drugs, 108
New Horizons, 64–5, 65f, 66f
NICE (National Institute for Health and Care Excellence), 151
Nigeria, attitudes to epilepsy, 35
Nightingale, Florence, 39
NIH (National Institute of Health), 176t
NIMH (National Institute of Mental Health), 72
NINDS (National Institute of Neurological Disorders and Stroke), 64
Nistico, Guiseppe, 62
non-disease effects of epilepsy, 8
Nootropil (piracetam), 176t

old (classic) antiepileptic drugs, 108
organisations, prescription of drugs, 151–2
orotracheal intubation, 104
Out of the Shadows (Global Campaign Against Epilepsy), 146, 147f, 176t
overdiagnosis, 119
over-medicalisation, 119
over-testing, 119
over-treatment, 120
oxazolidine diones, 49b
oxcarbazepine (Trileptal), 63f, 177t

paraldehyde, 174t
paroxysmal depolarisation shift (PDS), 6
partial seizures, generalised seizures *vs.*, 5
patients
  misleading by, 124–5
  subsets and antiepileptic drugs, 162
PDS (paroxysmal depolarisation shift), 6
Peck, Anthony W, 72
peer reviews, 140–1
Penfield, Wilder, 87–8, 88–9, 88f, 176t
Penry, J Kiffin, 62, 64
Penry, Kiffin, 53
pentylenetetrazole (PTZ) test, 68, 111
perampanel (Trobalt), 63f, 112, 178t
personality
  changes due to temporal lobectomy, 99
perceived personality faults, 25–6
PET (positron emission tomography), 93, 105
pharmaceutical industry, 54, 57–8
  ILAE, role in, 148–9
  mergers, 58–9
  power of, 54, 57
pharmacogenomics, 57–8
  alterations to antiepileptic drugs, 170
  phase I clinical trials, 57
  phase II clinical trials, 57
    gabapentin (Neurontin), 74
  phase III clinical trials, 57
    size and cost, 115
phenobarbital, 44–6, 66, 176t
  adverse effects, 44–5
  as controlled substance, 46
  depression, 109
  discovery, 44, 174t
  formularies, 46
  mechanism of action, 48
  societal history, 45–7
phenobarbitone, 58
phenytoin, 47–8, 66
  continuing use, 48
  first use, 177t
  introduction, 39
  mechanism of action, 48, 63f
  during pregnancy, 48
  status epilepticus, 175t
Philosophical Transactions of the Royal Society, 135
phrenological fallacy, 94–5, 96
physical nature of seizures, 6–7
piracetam (Nootropil), 176t
placebos
  controlled adjunctive trial design, 77
  delay in clinical trials, 114
  potential benefits, 165
Plan for Nationwide Action in Epilepsy, 176t
plant derivatives, 40–1, 41t
pleotherapy (multitarget treatments), 159
polypharmacy, 120
polytherapy, rational, 116
positron emission tomography (PET), 93, 105
postoperative psychiatric disturbances, 98–9
Post, Robert, 72
potassium bromide, 173t
potassium channels, 63f
pregabalin (Lyrica), 61, 66, 73, 75–6
  depression treatment, 109
  licensing, 177t
  mechanism of action, 63f
pregnancy
  antiepileptic drugs, 108
  phenytoin during, 48
  valproate, 53, 108
prejudice, societal attitudes, 33–4

premature mortality, 108–9
prescription of drugs, 151–2
presurgical assessment, 94, 103
prevention of epilepsy, 167–8
primidone (Mysoline), 175t
progabide, 62, 78
provocation by environmental factors, 132–3
psychoanalysis, 130–1
PTZ (pentylenetetrazole) test, 68, 111
publications *see* medical journals/publishing
PubMed (Medline), 142–3
Putnam, Tracy, 47, 175t

radiosurgery, 92
randomised controlled studies, temporal lobectomy, 98
random screening, antiepileptic drug discovery, 112
rare seizures, 110
rational polytherapy, 116
rattle-snake venom, 46
recapitulation, theory of, 129–30
recurrence of seizures, 170
refractory epilepsy *see* drug-resistant epilepsy (refractory epilepsy)
regulation *see* drug regulation
regulation of drugs *see* drug regulation
religious attitudes, 21
repurposing existing drugs, 159
Research Assessment Exercise, 142
resection *see* surgery
resistance to drugs *see* drug-resistant epilepsy (refractory epilepsy)
resolution of seizures in children, 155–6
retigabine/ezogabine (Trobalt), 63f, 112, 163, 178t
reviews, medical journals/publishing, 140
Reynolds, Edward, 71
Reynolds, John Russell, 175t
Rivotril (clonazepam), 176t
Rose, Hilary, 134–5
Rose, Steven, 134–5
rufinamide (Inovelon), 177t

Sabril *see* vigabatrin (Sabril)
Sagan, Carl, viii
Satzinger, Gerhard, 73–4
Saudi Arabia, attitudes to epilepsy, 35
Scherer, Hans Hoachim, 18
Schmidt, Bernd, 74, 79
Schmidt, Dieter, 64–5
science, technology and medicine (STM) journals *see* medical journals/publishing
scientific fallacy, 127
Scottish Intercollegiate Guidelines Network (SIGN), 151

Scully, Jackie, 10–11
sedation, phenobarbital, 45
SEEG (stereoelectroencephalography), 90, 175t
Seizure, 138
seizure diaries, 111
seizure-provocation tests, 111
seizures
    absence, 53
    cellular mechanisms, 6
    chemical nature of, 6–7
    chronic seizure tests, 112
    classification of type, 13
        Jacksonian seizures, 5
        myoclonic seizures, 53
        partial *vs.* generalised seizures, 5
        rare seizures, 110
        tonic–clonic seizures, 162
    definition of, 1, 3, 5–7
    development of, 94–5
    focal, 5
    freedom rates, 97
    physical nature of, 6–7
    recurrence of, 157, 170
    resolution in children, 155–6
    specific therapies, 162–3
    surgical outcomes, 97
seletracetam, 69
self-attitude to epilepsy, 36
self-publication, 142–3
sexuality post-surgery, 100–1
    post-temporal lobectomy, 99–100
Sieveking, Edward Henry, 22, 23f, 37, 40–1
SIGN (Scottish Intercollegiate Guidelines Network), 151
Simpson, James Young, 81
single-photon emission computed tomography (SPECT), 93, 105, 179t
single-target antiepileptic drugs, 159
6-Hz mouse test, 112
Skillman Village for Epileptics, 29
Smith, Richard, 135–6
Snow, John, 39
societal attitudes to epilepsy, 8–9, 21–35
    by country, 35
    definition of epilepsy, 16
    effects on science, 29
    epileptic and criminal characteristics, 25t, 26
    human rights, 34
    nineteenth century, 21–6
    perceived personality faults, 25–6
    phenobarbital, 45–7
    prejudice, 33–4
    stigmatisation, 36–7
    stigmatisation of epileptics, 36–7
    studies of, 34
    twentieth century, 26–37

sodium channels
  blockade, 58
  phenytoin mechanism, 48
Spatz, Hugo, 18
Special Marriage Act (1956), 33
SPECT (single-photon emission computed tomography), 93, 105, 179t
Spratling, William, 174t
statistics, 135
status epilepticus
  clonazepam (Rivotril), 176t
  phenytoin, 175t
stereoelectroencephalography (SEEG), 90, 175t
stereotactic surgery, 104
sterilization, 175t
stigmatisation of epilepsy, 36–7
stiripentol (Diacomit), 162, 177t
STM (science, technology and medicine) journals *see* medical journals/publishing
stroke, post-surgery, 98
structural abnormalities, 131–2
structural variants, antiepileptic drug discovery, 112
suboptimal doses, 121
sudden unexplained death in epilepsy (SUDEP), 109
  in clinical trials, 114
  tonic–clonic seizures, 162
suicidal ideation, 109
supersensitivity, 131
surgery, 81–106
  adverse effects, 98, 100–1
  anaesthesia, 81–2
  anterior temporal lobe resection, 176t
  antisepsis, 81, 104
  artificial demand, 102
  artificial demand of, 102
  awake craniotomy, 89
  congruent cases, 94
  corpus callosectomy, 91, 175t
  cortical resections, 86
  development of, 81–94
  EEG, 86–8
  electrical stimulation, 86
  'en bloc temporal lobe' resection, 89
  financial considerations, 101
  frontal lobectomy, 99
  frontal lobotomy, 99, 101
  functional hemispherectomy, 90–1
  functional maps, 83
  hemispherectomy, 90–1, 174t
  hippocampectomy of Yaşargil, 92
  ineffective procedures, 134b
  large frontal lobectomy, 99
  lesionectomy, 93
  mechanism of action, 95–6
  mortality, 98
  multiple subpial transection (Morrell procedure), 91–2, 177t
  outcomes of, 96–102
    anatomical area, 97
    cognitive changes after, 100–1
    potential benefits, 96
    seizure control, 97
  presurgical assessment, 94, 103
  regulatory approval, 97–8
  stereotactic surgery, 104
  technology assessment, 103
  temporal lobectomy *see* temporal lobectomy
  theoretical basis, 94–6
  unilateral temporal lobectomy, 99
  United Kingdom, 102
symptomatic zone, 95
symptoms, concealment of, 26, 28

Taiwan, 35
Talairach, Jean, 175t
Tallis, Ray, 134
target-based drug design, 112
target-related development of antiepileptic drugs, 158–9
taskforces, ILAE, 15–16, 145
Temkin, Owsei, 1, 2f, vii, 8
temporal lobectomy, 88, 89, 175t
  adverse effects, 98–9, 99–100
  randomised controlled studies, 98
  unilateral, 99
temporal lobe epilepsy (limbic epilepsy), 95–6
temporal lobes, 86
  functions, 98
thalidomide, 57, 152
theories of degeneration, 21–6, 129–30
theory of recapitulation, 129–30
tiagabine (Gabatril), 63f, 109, 112, 177t
tonic–clonic seizures, 162
Topamax *see* topiramate (Topamax)
topiramate (Topamax), 61, 66, 72–3
  adverse effects, 73
  depression, 109
  introduction, 179t
Traité de l'épilepsie (Delasiauve), 39–40
transcranial magnetic stimulation, 134
treatment, long-term, 120
The Treatment of Epilepsy, 55–6t
trial-and-error antiepileptic drug discovery, 112
triggering factors, 7
Trileptal (oxcarbazepine), 63f, 177t
Turner, W Aldren, 24, 42–3, 58, 174t

uncharacterised epilepsy, remission, 156f
uncomplicated epilepsy, remission, 156f
under-treatment, 121
unilateral temporal lobectomy, 99

United Kingdom (UK)
  attitudes to epilepsy, 35–6
  surgery, 102
Unverricht, Heinrich, 174t

valproate, 52–3, 66
  approval, 176t
  discovery, 176t
  introduction, 39
  pregnancy, 53, 108
variability of epilepsy, 107
video-telemetry electroencephalography, 90
vigabatrin (Sabril), 76
  adverse effects, 163
  depression, 109
  introduction, 177t
  mechanism of action, 112
  West syndrome, 162
Vimpat (lacosamide), 63f, 177t
viscosity, 24
voltage-gated sodium channel, 63f

Weeks, David, 29–30
Wegener, Friedrich, 18
Weissmann, Charles, 122
West syndrome, 162
Wilder, Russell, 174t
Workshops on Neurotransmitters in Epilepsy (WONOEP), 61–2
Workshops on the Determination of Antiepileptic Drugs in Body Fluids (WODADIBOF), 64
World Health Organization (WHO), definitions of epilepsy, 11–12
worldwide web, 138–9

Yuen, Alan, 72

Zarontin (ethosuximide), 47, 50, 63f, 175t
zinc, 46
Zola, Emile, 26
zonisamide (Excegran), 63f, 177t